You know deep down that the answer you are seeking is out there, you just haven't found it yet. You've tried so many weight loss programs. There is so much information available and yet, everything you have tried hasn't worked. I can tell you unequivocally today, that you have now found what you've been looking for! This is the last diet and weight loss book you will need in order to create that permanent change you long to enjoy. The average person once believed there was an answer to their weight problem, but gave up easily when they did not find it quickly. But you are not the average person! You never gave up searching for the answer. You don't give up easily. I hope you give the tools you receive in this book, a try, I hope you continue seeking for understanding until you discover what you have been searching for. I believe you'll find that what you have been seeking is right here in this book.

Weight Loss
ON THE GO

Simple ∞ Inspiring ∞ Permanent

Amy Twiggs

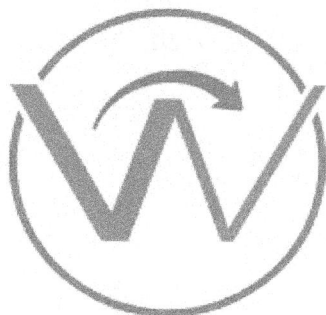

NOTICE

This book contains discussions about health issues and medical problems. While I have my own opinions about these topics, they are all just opinions based on my experience, training, and knowledge. I am not, nor pretend to be, a physician. If there are any questions about a medical concern, please refer to your primary-care physician or medical consultant. In addition, please be advised that I cannot be held responsible for medical decisions you make as a result of reading this book. Please contact your physician before undertaking any of the recommendations that I make.

AUTHOR'S NOTE

Throughout this book I have used examples from some of my clients' personal lives. However, to ensure privacy and confidentiality I have changed some of their names and some of the details of their experiences. None of the personal examples from my own life have been altered.

ISBN-13: 978-1-949015-07-2

ACKNOWLEDGEMENTS

Thank you, Tyler—I cannot say enough about how blessed I am to be married to him—I have known him since the 1st grade. He is a rock to everyone, especially me. He is steady and supportive and every time I get another crazy idea he gives me space to fulfill my dreams. I see him studying or watching "Adventure Time" with our kids and actually enjoying it and doing dishes night after night when I just want a "few more minutes on the computer." Tyler, you are exactly who I wanted and sometimes forget to appreciate. I sure love you.

To my amazing four teenagers who have always been patient with my "next lecture"—You encourage my words by sitting and commenting when I am seeking clarity. Thank you for being so self-reliant during those younger years, and still today. Thank you for being willing to entertain my morning idea of fun which, in the past, usually included practicing piano at 6:00 am and doing your chores before school, as I continued to work. You are such a source of joy and laughter and fulfillment in my life. I love watching each of you grow and teach me how to become better every day.

To my parents—You have always encouraged me. Everything I do is a highlight because of your excitement and involvement. You have always been my greatest fans. You have not only cheered me on during those years and years of gymnastics, but even now every day as I call to check in, you leave me with just enough love to keep me moving and learning as I endeavor to become as angelic as you both have always been.

To my clients—Thank you for your open-mindedness as you entertain new concepts and are willing to develop new habits in an effort to change your lives. My success comes in watching you achieve yours. Your enthusiasm and gratitude inspire me to continue striving to learn more and to share more. I am inspired every week by our coaching calls and our group sessions together. Thank you for making my life better in every way.

A FEW TESTIMONIALS

Now I have a greater understanding of why I crave the unhealthy foods that I do, and how to overcome those cravings. That understanding makes it easier for me to make healthier choices when it comes to food. Knowing what happens when you give in to your cravings, and understanding the false pleasure cycle, helps to remind me that I don't actually need those things my body is craving. I also really like the "Urge Worksheet." Visually seeing my urges helps me to have better control over them. This program is definitely a lot different than other programs I've tried. Most weight loss programs are just focused on diet and exercise, where this program is more educational and helps you to understand why weight loss has been an issue for you, and how to overcome it.

-McKayla Butcher

Before, I didn't realize it all started with thoughts. I was terrible to myself and didn't realize that it was projecting in my life. I'm starting my journey with the new information that gives me hope, with a different perspective that makes it easier to be more aware of how our thoughts and brain's works. Now I'm more motivated to really overcome the things that cause me to struggle with my weight as well as other things. I've noticed that I'm more motivated to improve my yoga poses and exercise daily to make any kind of movement in my life, because I want that energy to flow constantly with the help of my good thoughts. What really made me more aware is how Amy explained how our brain works with food. I had no idea that our brain has an impact on how we react to food. I'm more cautious with why and when or how I'm eating, and realize the difference between hunger for fuel vs. being conditioned to eat because that is how society has been doing it. I was extremely frustrated so I blamed it on my hypothyroid and tried to accommodate for that. I was diagnosed with primary lymph edema during that time, which explained why I was always so swollen but NOTHING seemed to work so I completely gave up, it became too hard especially not seeing any kind of results, so I let myself go. I tried other methods but I wasn't consistent. How Amy explained it from her weight loss point of view, I was like "OH!" I was missing the most important information in my previous journey. When Amy broke it down for me that it gave me a whole new perspective. I am more cautious of why I eat, and the tools were extremely helpful. The best part is it doesn't have to be hard.

-Meredith Poole

Before learning these tools I was very overwhelmed with life. I never felt like I had time to take care of myself because other things always took priority. However, as I am learning to apply the principles taught in this program I'm realizing that by making time for myself, everything else falls into place. No more guilt for taking care of me! :) Instead of worrying about what I'm eating, I think about how I'm feeling. This way of thinking has been extremely liberating. No more diets for me...ever!!! Throughout my entire life I have worried about my weight. It is such a relief to know that I don't have to think about what the number is going to be when I get on the scale. There is no number that will ever define me! This program isn't a diet...it's a way of life. The stress I used to feel about weight loss is gone. I just feel better!!

-Jana Wiltbank

As a stay at home mom with 5 young kids, I am often battling thoughts of doubt and discouragement. Being coached by Amy was nothing less than life-changing. The tools she gave me to truly believe I am enough and to feel the confidence I've been striving for have not only transformed me and the feeling in my home, but they are relevant to every other aspect of my life. Amy has an incredible amount of wisdom, and in 6 weeks of coaching calls was able to assist me in gaining the courage and the confidence I've been reaching for to create my life exactly the way I want it.

-Mindi Smith

Amy taught me to manage my thoughts and she explained why and how our minds work. It was mind blowing! Of all the weight loss programs I tried, this one is different and I can take the tools she taught me and keep my healthy weight stable. I have total control of what I eat and that is freedom! Food is now not my enemy.

-Missy Julien

I was so happy to find this training! Other weight loss programs will help you lose weight, but to keep it off you need to follow that plan for the rest of your life. I am not going to eat little packs of prepackaged food or count every calorie for the rest of my life. This is a lifestyle change and it's just what I have been looking for. This is something that you can do because you decide how to do it and you learn how to trust yourself in that process.

-Jennifer & Jordan Pusey

I've literally tried so many fad diets I've lost count! Obviously I wouldn't be even writing this if any of them had helped me with permanent weight loss. They were mostly quick fixes that promised results in 6 weeks or similar programs. I could not sustain the weight loss after I had lost the weight. The motivation was fueled by pure grit and determination, not anything permanent. I now have a whole new "toolbox" to help me with my permanent weight loss goals thanks to Amy Twiggs. She is a master at teaching this and I can't say enough about how happy I am with the results and life changing effects.

-Ellen Smedley

TABLE OF CONTENTS

INTRODUCTION

Want to STOP overeating? Are you addicted to sugar? Did you know that weight loss can be simple? Did you know that creating healthy eating habits isn't that hard? It's true!

What if weight loss didn't have to be hard! What if you were able to stop constantly thinking about food, sugar and your weight? What if that number on the scale was just a number and it had no sway over how you felt about yourself as a human being. What if you could enjoy the feeling of a permanent ideal weight just for you—the weight that would leave you energized, focused, healthy and feeling AMAZING in your summertime swimsuits!

Here's the truth--"by small and simple things are great things brought to pass; and small means in many instances doth confound the wise" (Book of Mormon, Alma 37:6) You want to know the simplest way to lose weight? Stop eating more than your body can use?

And here is the rest of an effective weight loss plan: Create a protocol that you are willing to commit to indefinitely.

Learn to trust yourself. Doing what you say you will do even when it's hard, is the most powerful skill that you can develop. Doing what you say you will do even if you don't want to, is the greatest part of self-confidence.

Self-confidence is having a firm trust in yourself and your abilities. It's your ability to trust yourself, knowing you can experience any emotion (including failure) without being harmed. Self-confidence is your overall opinion of yourself.

Who knew that losing weight had so much to do with self-confidence? And that weight loss was so simple? That's it. You can now close this book. You have been given the only two tips you need to successfully lose weight and keep it off permanently.

1. Eat less than your body can consume (don't eat more than your body needs).

2. Make a plan and stick to it.

It's as simple as that!

We think we want simple, but then our brains convince us that "it can't be that simple. There has to be more. It has to be harder."

What if it wasn't harder?

What if learning to trust yourself in any circumstance is all that there is to losing weight?
What if learning to have firm trust in ourselves is all there is to enjoyment in life and our weight really has nothing to do with everything else we want.

Maybe you think if you lose weight then you can feel happy and satisfied, comfortable and self-assured. What if that was a lie that kept you feeling inadequate and hesitant to live life to the fullest?

Think about it.

Knowing these tools is simple. Applying the tools takes consistent effort. If you want help applying the tools, that is my *superpower.* I will help you!

You join a fitness club, hoping to lose weight. You want to look good, but hesitate to go to those gyms because everyone around you ALREADY looks great. You feel embarrassed and inadequate. You wonder if you will ever have "their bodies."

Losing weight by exercise is possible, but eventually you realize that the kind of weight you want to lose will require much more than some yoga and kickboxing. It's the mental weight that pulls you down more than the physical weight.

After weeks of yoga and kickboxing, you find out that exercise alone, doesn't yield high weight loss results. Rather, exercise usually increases weight as you build muscle. Thus, you actually look bigger than when you started exercising.

You just want to feel healthy, strong, toned and energized. You don't want to have to worry about weight ever again, but are determined to do this one more time--hoping it's the last time. You are determined to make this last effort stick forever.

You tell yourself that this is the last "AFTER" picture! After an intense 6-12 week program, where you are starving, but seeing results, you take that "after program picture" to post on social media and feel proud of your accomplishments. You did it! You had the willpower to stick with that diet and exercise plan and finally felt the energy coming back and the self-acceptance increasing.

Then, somehow, those pounds started reappearing, unwelcome, but persistent. You thought, "It's no big deal...I know what to do...I'll start Monday to re-focus on those tools I learned in my last program. But for today, I will have this delicious chocolate cake with my best friend while she is in town. We deserve a treat and I have worked hard enough to enjoy one piece of cake." You eat that cake, then go home to realize you want another piece. Oh no! Now what?!

No big deal, you can start that intense program again when your life calms down a bit and your kids don't need you to take them everywhere or when the holidays are over and those treats are not all over the office tempting you.

This is a scenario that replays over and over. You can will-power your way through any weight loss program if you want to. But, what happens after that program? Why do you immediately revert to old habits? Why can't you stick to the diet plan that you paid so much money for?

I have been working to understand my weight issues since I was a nineteen-year-old at Stanford University on the women's gymnastics team. As a freshman, I tore my ACL doing a double back flip.

On my landing, my knee decided to go the wrong way. This was not a major problem as I was able to receive incredible help from Stanford doctors and therapy to get back to 100% activity by the following season.

Years later, I read that 95% of injuries to athletes in college are due to weight gain. Their bodies are not used to accommodating the extra weight.

Since that knee injury, I have struggled with my weight and body image. It's now been 23 years. I recall being told by nutritionists that I needed more fiber; or that I needed more iron; or I needed more steak, more protein, more fruit. But, do you know what I really needed?

I needed to understand, on a cognitive level, why I was eating what I was eating.

Most people believe that athletes can do anything. They are so strong, confident and happy. They overcome trials and appear to have superhero capabilities. I am not saying athletes are not amazing and focused. Athletes do overcome great feats. However, athletes are human.

Growing up, I did not come from a privileged home and our food selection was pretty plain and consistent. This was one of the greatest blessings of my life as an elite, National Team member.

However, when I went to college, the variety of food was limitless. That is when the lack of emotional education started to show its ugly face.

The amount of food provided at college was not monitored. The amount of weight gain was measured, not by my coaches, but by my performance. Weight gain was a natural consequence of an uneducated mind regarding food.

Sure, I could handle running extra miles after practice if I noticed my body start to change. I loved to exercise, so I assumed as long as I did more exercise, I would be able to keep up with my changing body weight. But, I did not keep up with my changing body because I didn't realize that my mind was a mess around food. The problem was my mind management, not the food.

To continue to perform at a high level, my beliefs regarding food were going to have to change. That was inevitable. I could have controlled my weight if I had known how to control my mind.

That is the oddest statement to confess. As competitive athletes, we are trained to manage our minds. I truly believed if I wanted to learn a new skill, I would learn it. I would practice the skill mentally and go to sleep doing visualization to understand how it might feel in my body-- the rhythm and power. Then I would try to apply that during practice. I was never nervous at even one meet in the four years of my college competition. I fell, but did not feel fear. Competing was a joy for me.

If my mind was so capable when it came to gymnastic skills and performance, why did I struggle to keep my mind strong around food? What was it about food that was so pleasurable and uncontrollable for me?

I majored in psychology with an added focus in health and development. I taught mental training and toughness for over fifteen years to hundreds of athletes and parents. Even with all those tools, I still struggled with my weight. I joined many fad diet programs and used will-power to succeed at each one. Just like you, I felt that I should be able to keep the weight off. I should not have had any issues with my weight because I had been taught the tools.

Logically, it's not that hard to lose weight. Why did I struggle so much to apply the knowledge? It wasn't until I became a certified Life and Weight Loss Coach through The Life Coach School that I finally understood what I was missing.

I am going to teach you the exact tools I now teach to my clients. They actually work.

These are tools that will help you not only get to your ideal weight, but keep the excess weight off forever. Then you can use these same tools, or meta-skills, if you want to change other areas of your life.

If you are anything like me, then you, too, may be tired of feeling like you should be smart enough to figure all of this out. Losing weight shouldn't be that hard. You wonder why you want those cookies or nachos so intensely that you give in, knowing you will regret it later.

You wish you had energy in the late afternoon, when your family needs you to be at your top level. You feel worn out, overworked, overwhelmed, frustrated, and ready to snap at anyone who asks anything more from you.

You just want to be able to slow down for a moment to get a bite to eat that will actually keep you fueled and moving instead of reaching for another handful of candy or that diet soda to keep your legs moving when your brain wants to go take a nap.

Maybe you think when your kids are older then you can take care of yourself and focus on your ideal healthy weight.

You believe when your life slows down, then you can create the health that will keep you hiking up those incredible mountains with your grandkids someday or go on that longed-for vacation with your husband.

Ideally, you don't want to worry about your weight or health when you are older, but you don't have time to take care of yourself right now so it will have to come later.

How can a life and weight loss coach help with these issues? What exactly is a weight loss coach and how can you benefit from having one?

Most clients just want to be told the exact steps to take, including the kinds and amounts of food, in order to get to that excess weight off as quickly as possible.

They believe that once they achieve their ideal weight, then their spouse will finally be romantic again, their kids will behave like normal human beings, their home will magically be organized, and all the stars will align to bring peace and harmony into their world.

These are the exact things that a life and weight loss coach addresses. A life and weight loss coach helps in every one of these areas: weight, relationships, money and lack of confidence— one thought at a time!

But for now, let's just start with that number on your scale.

The weight issue requires one small skill that will trickle into every other area of your life.

Once you become a self-coaching master regarding your current weight issues, you will find the rest of your life won't seem so overwhelming, frustrating, and out of control.

If you have never had a life and weight loss coach, you have been missing out! It's like being told that you need a smartphone and you wonder why you would want that.

You cannot know the power that the phone has until you get one and try out the functions. Then you realize that you don't know how you ever lived without one.

That is exactly what a life and weight loss coach is. It's your secret "smartphone" just waiting to be discovered. You will never be the same again.

I've written this book after the same pattern I use for my clients that come seeking individual coaching help. This book is focused specifically on weight loss.

However, it doesn't matter what kind of help you need. The coaching tools apply to every area of your life. We start in Phase I with the simplest, yet most powerful tool towards reaching lifestyle goals. Then, Phase II covers what you think you want, which is a specific step by step weight loss plan.

In Phase III, we focus on mind management education, food protocol principles and then more mind management tools.

Yup, you heard that right! Mind management is to permanent weight loss like water is to the body. You cannot go very long without your mental hydration. Otherwise, you will feel mental dehydration, that always results in a loss of focus, energy, and control.

You will start to realize as you progress through this program, that there are so many more issues going on beneath the weight loss concern.

You will rediscover your dreams, your passions and your goals. **The mental tools provided, will lead you to the life that you always wanted, but did not know how to find.**

This book will provide the answer to your question about how to actually lose weight permanently. You do not have to feel like you are on a hamster wheel when it comes to dieting ever again. When you learn the cognitive science behind your actions with food, then you will understand why you do what you do and can change it.

Awareness is always the first step to every change. If we don't know, then we won't ask. If we don't ask, then we won't find answers. Self-understanding is a process and one worth taking time to uncover.

If you apply the tools that I teach in this book, you will not only create permanent weight loss, but can use these meta-skills to change anything you want in your life. I am so thrilled for you to have this book and I hope it brings you much satisfaction now and in your future endeavors.

The way I've organized this book is for you to first, have something you can run with immediately for weight loss success. Then, you will be given a specific food protocol plan if you want one. The final phase includes background education so that you can understand the WHY of the WEIGHT.

Since we all want instant gratification (which means that our brains are working perfectly and nothing is wrong with us), I will give you a quick sneak peek now, at the FOOD PROTOCOL that you will find in Phase III.

This sneak peak is for busy people, not for people who actually want to read an entire book before getting to the *meat* of the topic. This way, if you decide not to wait for more information, then you have something you can run with now and still be very successful.

Sneak Peak at Phase III:
After-AFTER Magic Formula Summarized

Chapter 3: 5 Pillars to Personal Permanent Weight Loss, includes:

Pillar #1   Time Window: Decide when you will start and when you will stop eating for the day.

Pillar #2   What to Eat: What types of foods are best for you? You decide.

Pillar #3   How much to Eat: How much food at each sitting will you consume?

Pillar #4   When to Eat: How often within that time window will you eat?

Pillar #5   Documentation & Planning: Record, Record, Record. Plan. Plan. Plan. Wait 2 weeks, then tweak only ONE of the first four pillars until you find the perfect protocol for your body. Continually ask yourself, "How do I feel?" and "Why?" This last pillar is crucial for any permanent change.

The application of these 5 pillars are all about building personal confidence.

Phase I

All You Need To Know

No More Excuses! Let's make weight loss as simple as it gets. There is only one tool you need for permanent weight loss. Here is it: **Make a plan and commit to it!** Sound simple? It is! Learning something is easy. Teaching you how to apply the knowledge is my personal superpower!

That's it! You can now close this book if you feel satisfied and ready to apply Phase I to your life. Go on to Phase II if you seek more help and understanding.

Phase II

Before & After: What You Think You Want

We all want to be given a specific plan to follow. A predetermined plan makes it easy to know what to try based on the success of many other people.

"It's not about perfect. It's about effort. And when you bring that effort every single day, that's where transformation happens. That's how change occurs."

-Jillian Michaels

"Take care of your body. It's the only place you have to live."

-Jim Rohn

Here is the part where I tell you exactly what to do to lose those stubborn last 10 pounds or those first 50 pounds. The process is the same. The third phase of this book will provide you the tools to keep those pounds off. But, for now, let's DO the action required to get the weight off, the results you want. In three months, you'll thank yourself.

Most people use willpower to get through these first 12 weeks feeling like they are torturing themselves and miserable. They will continue to push through in order to know they really can accomplish hard things and create a healthier body in the process.

Is this sustainable? Maybe. But, there is a deprivation-free way to keep the pounds off for good that will be unveiled soon. In Phase III, I will teach you how to keep the results you work so hard to create.

Right now, I will give you the exact steps to get to the "after" picture we all enjoy so much. You will be able to frame that one!

First, a quick story. I recall supporting a friend on a diet. I had a few pounds that I wanted to lose, so I agreed to join in on one of my friend's latest fad diets. She had 2 more days left and if she lost 5 more pounds, she could get her $500.00 deposit refunded. It was a challenge that she had accepted 10 weeks earlier, but didn't realize how soon her will-power would dwindle. While I was visiting her on a vacation, we took our kids to parks and rivers and movies. Between the two of us, we had 10 kids. It was a load. And they got hungry often.

We had to pre-plan for the children's food and for our food separately. It was actually pretty simple to plan our food as my friend chose to pack tilapia and asparagus for our three meals every day. By the last day, I wasn't sure that I ever wanted to look, smell, or eat fish again. I forced myself to down it in an effort to support my friend, but I have not touched tilapia again since. What kind of lifestyle is that?

I used to enjoy tilapia, but now I cannot stand the thought of it. If I had the tools then that I have now, I might eat tilapia again. But, that is still a food that I don't choose to eat.

My friend did lose the five pounds she needed and got her money back, but she soon gained the weight right back once "the challenge" was over.

Can you relate? Have you ever forced yourself to complete a challenge just to return to your old habits? Does this make you want to try another 12-week plan? If you are saying to yourself, "It's not worth the effort again," then just know that your brain is working perfectly. This book will teach you a new approach to healthy weight loss. You are going to be learning tools and gaining skills that will not leave you feeling disappointed and disgusted with yourself. Are you ready for a new life? Are you ready to commit to yourself and create new neural pathways that will empower you and obliterate the over-desire for food and sugar? Then, let's get started!

You are now ready to learn the 12 simple steps for your 12-week weight loss program.

Here they are:

1. Take a "Before" picture.

2. Drink enough water to equal half your body's weight (i.e., 100 lbs = 50 oz water). If you engage in exercise, you will want to add half a teaspoon of sea salt to every quart of water in order to replace electrolytes.

    a. In general, water needs will change based on activity and seasons of the year/temperature. Drinking 64 ounces or half your body's weight (in ounces) is recommended by many doctors. In order to make the process easy, I suggest you buy a few of your favorite extra-large water bottles. Keep one in your car, in the kitchen, next to your bed, and anywhere else you find yourself stopping often. If you keep your car cup holders filled with water bottles, then you will be less likely to use those cup holders for extra-large soda pops. Be sure to refill and replace the water bottles daily.

3. Pack two containers of vegetables with your favorite healthy dip.

    a. Guacamole, hummus, and bean dips are great options. Try adding different vegetables during the program. I would encourage you to have these prepared every night for the following day.

b. Vegetable options (eat at two meals/day): broccoli, asparagus, carrots, cauliflower, green beans, bell peppers, mushrooms, spinach, tomato, peas, cabbage, celery, zucchini, cucumber, onion, brussel sprouts, artichoke, lettuce or other vegetables of your choosing.

c. Side note: you can repeat steps one-three for the next 12 weeks and obtain great results. See what happens! It can't get much more simple. Water and vegetables are the two things most people need to add to their food plan to gain initial traction on a permanent weight loss journey. Our brains do not like to feel deprived! *Adding* food to our normal eating habits feels doable and non-threatening. If you want to continue to see quicker results, then move on to the next steps.

4. Get rid of all the snack foods in your home and car—including those hidden snacks for those "hangry" or "stressful" moments, that are stashed away under your driver seat. Snacks are never necessary.

5. Pre-plan to eat one meal per week that is off the food plan. I call this a Joy Eat. It's to be guilt-free and thoroughly enjoyed!

6. Pre-plan one fast of 2 meals during the 12-week weight loss program. Try to skip two meals or go 24 hours with no food or water if possible—remember that this is a suggestion and I am not a doctor! The benefits of intermittent and periodic fasting are worth it if your body can handle it. I encourage you to search the benefits of fasting online and decide for yourself.

7. Choose 1 of the following eating plans:

- Plan A:
  a. Eating times: 6:00am, 8:30am, 11:00am (include a pre-planned vegetable pack), 1:30pm, 4:00pm (include a pre-planned vegetable snack), 6:30pm

  b. Food selection: You can mix and match your own choices or choose from the list that is provided in the next step.

  c. Amount of food: At each meal, one serving of protein and carbohydrates based on the recommended values that you can find printed on the back of any packaged food.

- Plan B:
  a. Eating times: 6:00am, 12:00pm (include a pre-planned vegetable snack), 6:00pm (include a pre-planned vegetable pack)

b. Food selection: You can mix & match your own choices or choose from the list that is provided in the next step.

c. Amount of food: At each meal, choose one-two servings of protein and carbohydrates based on recommended values that you can find printed on the back of any packaged food.

8. Food selection options: These are just recommendations. You can choose your own, but keep them similar to these types of foods for the first 6 weeks.

- Protein: Chicken breast, turkey breast, lean ground beef, tuna, salmon, crab, lobster, shrimp, top round steak, top sirloin steak, lean ham, eggs, cottage cheese, ricotta cheese, cheese, tofu, unsweetened almond milk, plain yogurt, beans, hummus, lentils, nuts, veggie burger, soy nuts or edamame

- Carbs: baked potato, sweet potato, yam, squash, steamed brown rice, steamed wild rice, pasta, oatmeal, oat bran, quinoa, millet, fiber one, cream of rice, rice, shredded wheat, grits, beans, strawberries, melon, apple, orange, yogurt, milk

- Good fats: butter, nut butter, olive oil, avocado oil, avocado, mayonnaise, salad dressing (no sugar), seeds, olives, peanut oil, other nut oils, heavy cream, sour cream

- Alright to have: Condiments, broths, spices

- Up to you: Dark chocolate, artificial sweeteners

- Avoid: Anything with flour, sugar, trans fats, processed, concentrated, and refined foods

9. Repeat steps one through eight for 12 weeks.

10. Take an "After" picture.

   Keep the Before & After picture together.

   Post the pictures somewhere where you can see them often. This does not necessarily mean on social media. Just post them where you can see the progress you have made as a daily reminder.

11. Get a food tracker app on your phone or a notebook to track your food intake.

12. Get a scale. Weigh yourself daily. Track and analyze data. Look for patterns.

Here are a few extra items you may want to include, daily, as you begin a lifestyle transformation. These are optional. However, they have been shown to increase energy and satisfaction in life:

- Sunlight daily (recommended 20-30 minutes)

- Sleep (recommended 7-9 hours depending on age)

- Fun (you choose)

- Connection (spend time interacting with other people face-to-face)

- Exercise (20-30 minutes)

Do not go any further until you have completed Steps 1-12 for 12 weeks... unless you want to.

CONGRATULATIONS!

You have built some amazing skill sets in Phases I & II in order to get to this point!

Now, go to Phase III to learn how to maintain the "after" picture.

Phase III

After-AFTER: Making It Last

What you really want...is to keep the weight off forever.

"Change your thoughts, change your world."
-Norman Vincent Peale

CHAPTER ONE

Obstacles

"Obstacles don't have to stop you. If you run into a wall, don't turn around and give up. Figure out how to climb it, go through it, or work around it."

-Michael Jordan

The Basics

"I'm so freakin' fat." This was said by a client recently. I asked her how it felt to believe that she was *"freakin' fat,"* She responded, *"miserable and sad."* When she feels miserable, my client said she eats cookies and then she continues to be *"freakin' fatter."*

What if I tell you that her brain was doing exactly what it was programmed to do? She was responding to life perfectly.

There is another way, however. You just have to know why your brain does what it does, in order to change what you do. Losing weight is not about the number on the scale, it has to do with your thoughts about the number on the scale. When you understand those belief systems that are creating your current weight, and why you hold onto those beliefs, then the real magic of permanent weight loss begins.

The question is: Why are you overweight? The answer is very simple. You are overweight because you eat more food than your body needs. If this principle is all you need to know, and if you understand this completely, then there should be no overweight issues, right?!

I mean, look around, the facts are everywhere. If you want to learn "how to eat for a healthy body," you only need to type that phrase into the search engine of any computer and you will see that a plethora of knowledge is readily available to everyone.

So, why, with all this information, are there still an overwhelming number of weight issues running rampant throughout our country? It is easier and takes less energy, to NOT pick up a spoon and put that scoop of ice cream into your mouth than it is to pick it up and eat with it.

These concepts are easy to understand. You can lose weight and keep it off permanently when you learn why you think about food in the way that you do. I will show you what I mean.

In this section, I am not going to pretend to know all the answers to every person's weight issues. I will be talking in generalities, using a broad spectrum of overall research. I will give you the tools I teach and you are welcome to use them, believe them, enjoy them, or toss them. You always have a choice.

You always get to do whatever you want and that is one of the amazing facts about being human! You have free agency. Nobody can tell you what to do or how to live or what will make you feel like you are enough as a human.

The privilege of being human provides you with the ability to challenge every thought that your brain offers you. Because you are human, you can create a whole new experience in your life in an intentional and beautiful way.

Evolution

Let's start with human evolutionary psychology. Did you know that your brain is pre-wired to do three specific things, namely, avoid pain, seek pleasure and use very little energy. This is called the motivational triad and it has kept our species alive for thousands of years.

This motivational triad was very important when humans needed to find shelter and search for food to survive. However, today, most of us have constant shelter and plenty of food, or at least know where we can go to get some.

Resources are plentiful. There is very little lack in our country. What the motivational triad, or the evolutionary software that has been downloaded into your brain looks like is you sitting on a couch, eating your favorite ice cream and watching Netflix.

This keeps you safe, uses very little energy and provides plenty of "pleasure." I will talk about insatiable versus satisfying pleasure later on. But for now, you just need to understand that this is exactly what your brain has evolved to do for you.

When you want to sit down, grab that quick fast food item or those handfuls of candy and chips at 3:00 pm and just relax, then you can know that your brain is working perfectly. You are not lazy or undisciplined. You are human, allowing your primitive brain to function exactly the way it is programmed.

This kind of life, today, does not actually serve us well. When we continue to allow our brain to tell us what is most important, then we will eventually discover that our lives are unsatisfying. A hedonistic person lives basically from the motivational triad.

This type of person believes that pleasure is the most important thing in life and pursues immediate pleasure above any long-term satisfaction.

Is this lifestyle wrong? Who am I to say that no person should live this way? I am not a judge of what someone should or shouldn't do. I make plenty of choices that others may believe are not productive or useful. I will not attempt to tell you what you should and shouldn't do— not even in the "diet plan" that I will be offering later on in this book.

You will always be the best and only person that can decide what you should do for you.

However, I will offer suggestions based on my clients' experiences and my own. I have learned from personal experience that when I allow my primitive brain to run the show, I am left wanting.

Your brain always seeks ways to help you survive, which is its primary job. But your indomitable, divine spirit wants deeper meaning and purpose in life.

As I apply the opposite of the motivational triad in my life, I feel fulfilled, challenged and satisfied beyond imagination.

What does this mean? What is the opposite of the motivational triad?

Instead of avoiding pain, seeking pleasure and using very little energy, you need to challenge that evolved brain that has kept you and your ancestors alive for so long. This means you will want to do something for personal growth rather than only historically-based survival.

This is the new Modern Motivational Triad, as taught by master coach, Brooke Castillo:

1. Seek Growth

2. Embrace Discomfort

3. Expend Massive Effort Wisely

You will feel like the little chick trying to come out of that eggshell. If that chick stays in the shell, he/she will die. If he/she doesn't expend effort and work hard, he/she will realize no growth, no healthy life, no true evolution.

Like the chick, our evolved brain must once again evolve into something it has never experienced before. This will require discomfort and effort.

The more willing we are to feel uncomfortable, the more guaranteed we will be to achieve our desired long-term results. Does that mean we must feel uncomfortable forever? No! Only when we want worthwhile change in our lives—no problem, right!

Here is a tip to help you survive the new triad: **You are capable of experiencing any emotion, including discomfort, without being harmed.**

Environment

One of the biggest weight loss lies we try to untangle in our brains is the lie that society tries to feed us which is, that there must be something wrong with us if we don't eat dessert and at the same time maintain a thin body.

Those two environmental beliefs are contradictory. Most humans cannot eat whatever they want whenever they want and maintain a size two body type.

And yet, if they do not remain thin, they might be judged by others.

You go to that family dinner and when the dessert comes around, if you don't partake of the goodness to acknowledge the effort behind the beautiful meal, you might feel selfish.

You have to make excuses to feel justified, and more often than not, you will agree to just a "small slice." Then, you go to that pool party a week later and feel uncomfortable and embarrassed by that extra weight on your thighs and wonder who else is staring at your imperfect figure, thinking you should really get back on that diet because there is some work to do. How is this okay?

How is anyone supposed to feel successful if this is what we are trained and conditioned to believe is normal. And what is normal? Is this normal? Who decided that we have to look alike and fit the same mold in order to feel good about ourselves and to fit into the societal circles of acceptable people?

We either feel like there is always something wrong with us, or we are missing out on life if we are not capable of fitting in with the societal norms.

Where is the peace if society says there is no way you will win? How do you find a way to "fit in" when there is no "fitting in"? All entertainment typically revolves around food.

We have trained ourselves and each other to believe that we must eat more than we need, we must eat when others are eating, and we must eat all day long.

The world says, it is socially acceptable to act in these ways and socially awkward when we don't.

Here is a tip to help with this issue: **You are not the world!**

Your Brain

Let's talk about your brain. Based on the motivational triad that we just discussed, we are now able to understand better why we resist change. Change requires effort.

Effort is an inefficient manner of living according to our primitive brain. One pillar of that old motivational triad, is using as little energy as possible. This is wise, to conserve energy for a time when we really need it.

Those moments happen rarely in our lives, but your brain does not know this. It wants to be prepared for those tigers that might jump out and start chasing you at any time.

The tigers most of us are running from these days are created only in our minds. But, your primitive brain does not know the difference between the real tiger and a mental tiger (better known as any negative feeling).

Ninety-five percent of the time, the neurological programming is very useful. It's the other 5% that causes so much suffering and discontent in our lives.

A habit, which is just doing an action over and over, is an efficient way to live. Your habitual food choices (amounts and types) are efficient. In order to create a new habits, there will have to be some discomfort as you work counter to your brain's evolved tendency.

Creating new habits will not feel efficient until you have repeated an action enough times that you teach and train your brain to make your new way (your new neurological pathways) efficient, and therefore, form a new habit.

Many habits are helpful, (i.e., walking, driving, cleaning, brushing your teeth). These types of activities we want to delegate to our subconscious brain so we don't have to consciously think about each step of the process.

When we drive a direction from work to our home enough times, we may experience thoughts such as, "huh, I don't even remember what happened between work and home." Our brain was being very efficient and allowing us the privilege of thinking of other things as we drove the worn physical and neurological pathway to our home.

This is exactly what we do with ANY habit we have. When we repeat the action enough times those actions are delegated to the subconscious in an effort to conserve energy for other, more important issues at hand.

But, what if our highly efficient habits are not always helping us survive? What if our brain is confused about which habits will help and which ones will hurt us in the long run? This is one of the challenges we get to enjoy as humans.

You get to decide when the neurological pathways that you have created need to be tweaked and redirected to become more useful. Whenever you decide to make a change, you are also deciding on an inefficient and inevitably, uncomfortable new pathway which will require work and planning and development.

New pathways, just like with new roads, will take time and effort. It will feel difficult and "inefficient." However, it is the only way to create a new path. You must plan for the brain to say, "Wait! The old road was perfectly fine! Why do you have to mess with what you already established to be a great path? This does not feel good. Make a U-turn, recalibrate, you are going into the unknown, you might die!"

If your brain does this, or more likely it will be "when" your brain offers these ideas, you can know that your brain is working perfectly and you are on the right path! Just keep going!

Your lower brain is what I like to call your primitive or survival brain. I have heard it called your downstairs brain, lizard brain, and part of your limbic system. I use these terms interchangeably.

It houses your amygdala, which is where your intense emotions are initiated. Now remember, I am not pretending to say that I know much, but I know enough to help you rewire your brain so that food is something you can enjoy as a lifelong friend instead of that "friend" that stabs you in the back as soon as you walk away.

Here is a tip to help with your survival brain: **You are not your brain!**

Biology
This section has similarities to the brain information, but with some different twists.

Biology includes the study of behavior. If you want to understand why so many people are overweight, the answer is easy.

They eat too much. But why?

It's, in part, because our brains are designed to be rewarded for survival activities. Food helps us survive. The reward we feel when we eat comes from many chemicals that are released into our bodies.

A few of these chemicals include dopamine, endorphins, oxytocin, and serotonin. These chemicals may feel good, or help us feel connected to others, or give us a desire and energy to take some action. They are useful and necessary for enjoyment in our lives.

We look for cues that create neural pathways to remind us of how great it felt the last time we ate something and how important it must be for us to get some more food again and again.

Most people know what foods to eat and what foods will not serve them in the long run.

Most of us know that when we eat too much, our pants will eventually "shrink" and feel tight.

The best advice you often hear is to eat only when you are hungry. But then you go to a social event and are asked why you're not eating. We've talked about societal norms that create some discord in weight issues.

What really matters is your thoughts about food and weight loss. The thoughts that you have rehearsed over and over to create your thought errors (non-useful belief systems), in an attempt to be efficient, are what is holding you back from achieving success--that is what your brain wants. But remember, you are not your brain.

All the food industries in our country conduct their marketing based on taking advantage of our desire for pleasure with using very little energy. This has created an over-desire for foods that can actually harm you instead of sustaining life.

One way to combat this effort by the food industry is through the knowledge obtained in the field of psychology. We must learn to manage our emotions around food using cognitive-based tools.

Most people do not know how to cope with the variety of instant pleasures all around them. If we can educate our country to improve individual emotional and mental management, then the potential for creating extraordinary lives will become limitless.

We can stop feeling stuck, trapped and out of control. Rather, we can feel capable, empowered, and confident in our ability to override our survival brain.

Here is a tip to help with your biology: **You have free agency, use it!**

CHAPTER TWO

Causes of Overweight

*"The abundance of cheap food with low nutritional value in
the Western diet has wreaked havoc on our health;
in America, one third of children and two thirds
of adults are overweight or obese and are
more likely to develop diabetes and
cardiovascular disease".*

-Ellen Gustafson

The Overweight problem in our country has to do with two
foundational issues:

1. Over-hunger

2. Over-desire

If we could solve both of these issues, then there would be
very few obesity concerns.

Over-hunger
Let's first solve the over-hunger problem, then we can
tackle the over-desire issue.

If you understand a bit about a few hormones that impact
your food consumption, then you will begin to see why it's
so easy to fall prey to over-hunger. There are three main

hormones to look at when it comes to weight gain or weight loss.

The most important hormone involved in our weight is insulin. Most obesity is caused by too much insulin in the blood. Insulin is a fat storage hormone, so whenever it is elevated in the blood, the body cannot burn or utilize fat as fuel.

Insulin, insulin resistance, and diabetes have skyrocketed with the increase in production and consumption or high sugar and high starch foods. Insulin also affects the presence and effectiveness of the hormones, leptin and ghrelin.

Leptin is a hormone in the body that lets us know when we're full and don't need to consume any more food. It also lets us know when it's time to move on. However, it's blocked in the brain by an excess of insulin, which means that we don't know when we are full. This is why we can consume a lot of processed foods and not feel full. Our brain is not able to tell the body that it has had enough food.

The other hormone that is useful to understand a bit about in our weight loss education is called Ghrelin. This hormone is also known as the "hunger hormone." This hormone is found in the gastrointestinal tract or the gut, and it simply lets us know when we're hungry. It's affected negatively by concentrated foods because it doesn't recognize the caloric intake of those types of food.

Why do we need to know this? So that we can be more aware of what is happening inside our bodies and our brain when we consume concentrated foods. This knowledge may help us choose to take different actions that will serve us better. Concentrated foods are foods consisting of flour, sugar and other manmade, processed foods.

When you have the physical sensation of hunger, your body is telling you that it needs some fuel to continue performing at a satisfactory level. So physical hunger is a sensation from the body that moves to the brain to remind you to get food.

When you actually are hungry, you might feel waves of hunger that come and go. If you don't eat right away, you will use fat for fuel. Over-hunger is caused by hormone imbalance, cravings and withdrawal. We all know exactly how much to eat. Our bodies are amazing at providing information if we choose to listen and if we keep our receptors open to receive the information.

When you eat natural foods, your body knows what to do. Hormones remain balanced easier and hunger signals are clear. However, we have conditioned ourselves to crave artificially concentrated foods that our bodies struggle knowing how to process.

The goal is always to reduce your hunger so you are only hungry for the very small amount of food your body actually needs. When you are not eating all the time, then your body can access your fat stores. This is called being fat adapted.

When you are really trying to lose weight, you want to use these fat stores as one of your main sources of fuel. How do you know when you are fat adapted? Fat adaptation is manifest when you are able to go 12-16 hours easily without food. If you eat all the time, then you will not become fat adapted.

When you feel like quitting, remember why you started this journey in the first place.

You brain will want you go back to feeling comfortable taking the easy road. That is not as satisfying as knowing what you are capable of. When you feel like quitting, just know that is exactly what your brain is supposed to offer you at this point.

Over-desire
The second reason people are overweight has to do with over-desire for food.

<u>Conditioning</u> (how we create habits)
Let's talk about Pavlov's dogs. When I was at Stanford University, I can recall sitting in a large lecture hall learning about Pavlov, a great behavioral scientist who is well known today for his study of dogs and the neurotransmitter, dopamine.

Dopamine is a chemical released by the brain that motivates us to act. When talking about dopamine, many life coaches use the phrase, "it gives you a dopamine hit" to mean your brain really wants more of something due to the intense release of this chemical and it will seek out cues for more of what caused that chemical to be released.

So, for instance, when you eat a donut and your insulin levels increase quickly, your brain thinks, "Wow, that was amazing, that felt good, I should get more of those donuts. I must be important to my survival!"

The dopamine released comes from our thoughts, and it causes us to seek more and more and more of those kinds of foods. Every time we answer those thoughts or cravings, the deeper that road or neurological pathway becomes and the easier it is for us to turn to donuts as a life sustaining food rather than veggies that do not increase insulin quickly and, therefore, do not release dopamine as dramatically.

Our brain avoids pain and seeks pleasure. Donuts make us feel good, but the results are not sustaining. Our survival brains do not understand the difference. Those repeated thought patterns get us every time.

So, what do we learn about Pavlov and dopamine? Pavlov, in a brief summary, had a group of dogs. He would ring a bell, and the dogs would come to eat food.

This activity was repeated: bell, food, bell, food. Pavlov noticed something interesting. After repeating this action for some time, as soon as he would ring the bell, the dogs started to salivate before they got the food. What was happening?

They were experiencing enjoyment of the reward without actually having the reward. How can that be? When they actually got the reward, which is the food, the dopamine levels stopped.

The actual reward was no longer releasing dopamine. It was the thought, the expectation of the reward, that released the dopamine, which motivated the dogs to move towards the food.

What does this information do for us? Well, if you have expected yourself to act in a certain way for a long time, and if you have trained your brain to believe that breakfast is at 9:00 am, lunch is at noon, dinner is at 6:00, then dessert closes your day, what happens when you miss breakfast? Then lunch?

Your brain starts to freak out. You start to drool and salivate. By dinner, your brain wants you to believe that you have got to eat and eat and eat as fast as you can, otherwise you might die!

You have deprived yourself and that was not safe nor enjoyable. It required a lot of energy because you were thinking about when your next meal would come. This is not an efficient way of living based on your brain's standards.

We condition ourselves to believe that some routines and habits are important for survival. What if this isn't the case at all? What if you could challenge that primitive brain and wait for your body to feel hunger?

That would be different right? And different requires energy. And that is not efficient, so we lapse back into the most efficient routines of our past to keep us surviving in the future. If you've survived this long, then why change now?

A better question is, why not change? What are your habits creating in your life? Some are useful, but what about those habits that you believe are important that may not be useful—the 5% of default thoughts that are not useful for survival?

Moms are amazing! They sacrifice and sacrifice and give and give. If I ask clients that are moms about taking a little time for self-care, what do you think they say? "Oh, well, when my kids are gone maybe," or "there's just too much to do to stop and focus on myself."

The only problem with these thought patterns is that if you don't take care of yourself, then you will wish you had in the future when you are limited by health issues that could have been prevented.

We all like instant gratification. Society seeks out sugar, flour, alcohol, porn, busy, work, gossip, social media and drugs. These provide immediate "dopamine hits." It feels good to seek more of these things, even if they could kill us.

I wonder if busy moms sacrificing their health and time get just as much instant gratification in an insatiable manner as other addicts do from their choice of addiction?

Maybe the consequences are not as apparent as someone who smokes, but in the long run, maybe they are. Mom's want to feel like they are contributing, serving, and doing their best. Serving others appears on the outside to be life sustaining, purposeful, and contributing. And it is... until it isn't.

When it causes us to neglect these amazing bodies (also referred to as "temples") that we have been given to care for, don't you think it is worth considering that taking care of ourselves, our bodies and our minds might just be one of the best ways to take care of our families and communities in the long-term? Serving from a place of inner-peace, unconditional self-love, and physical and emotional health will provide a lot more energy to serve others and love others unconditionally. Our ability to love others is based on our ability to feel love. If we neglect ourselves, what kind of service can we sustain long-term?

When we judge another person for their addiction, we don't have to look far to find our own. And again, each addiction carries its own consequences, some more apparent and damaging than others. I know clients don't like to compare their sugar or food addictions to drug addictions. There are definitely differences, but there are also some similarities. Both have created pathways in the brain that are on auto-pilot and do not serve the body. Both are generating false pleasure and both are satisfying an immediate desire.

When we agree with our survival brains, then we are using old thought patterns that play like a bad re-run over and over. What we think about creates our results. If we continue to eat non-useful foods, then we are allowing our primitive brain to win. We are using default settings when we could have a much more satisfying life experience!

So, if we are the cause of all our problems, how do we stop causing them?

De-conditioning (how to break unwanted habits)

One of the best parts of Pavlov's experiment is that he showed how a dog is conditioned to respond with drool without even receiving the reward. The dog actually gets the reward of dopamine, which feels motivating and pleasurable, before he/she gets food.

I have talked about how we, too, do this with food. The idea of dinner begins a dopamine release and it doesn't go away until you answer that desire with food. Then the dopamine stops.

So, to de-condition yourself from food that doesn't serve you, do what Pavlov did. Stop giving yourself the reward. What? No food? No treats, donuts, soda, pick your favorite. This is not what I am saying. But, if you truly want to break a habit that is creating negative results in your life, the solution is actually very simple.

You stop doing it. Use your free agency and choose to stop. But, that seems harder than actually continuing the bad habit. Why?

Pavlov watched his dogs constantly drool before they got food. Then he decided to stop putting the food out. The dogs would hear the bell ring, start to drool (get that dopamine hit), run for the food, and look for a reward that just wasn't there.

They went away disappointed and deprived. Did you know that disappointment and deprivation are just emotions in the body? They can never hurt you and will not kill you.

Do you want to feel them? Most of us avoid or resist these kinds of emotions at all costs. We will even eat day old french fries left on the counter from last night's fast food run in order to avoid feeling deprived. "Well at least the kids didn't eat all the food, they left me a few fries." Right?!

This is what we think. And somehow we feel a tinge of emotional relief with these terrible food leftovers.

Pavlov's dogs continued to drool and drool. In fact, the drool increased as the reward continued to not be there when they came running. Then, one day, all of the sudden, the drool stopped.

Does that mean they stopped wanting food? No! The dopamine stopped being released because it was a waste of energy. And our primitive brains do not like to waste energy.

There was no point in releasing energy running for something that would not be there. They still wanted it, but the over-desire that was conditioned and apparent by the dopamine and drool, was now gone. They no longer expected a reward and therefore stopped running for the food.

This is exactly what we need to do, and will want to learn how to do, in order to stop the over-desire that our evolution, our society, our brains and our biology have combined to work on within us. It's a simple process really. It just takes diligence and awareness.

An Urgent Desires Worksheet is included at the end of this section. Basically, you write down 100 urges, urgent desires, or cravings you have for food, or anything else (such as complaining, gossiping, social media, porn, alcohol, drugs) that you do not answer-- no expected reward after the drool.

You can use this simple, but extremely powerful, tool to de-condition yourself from expecting to react immediately to your non-useful urgent desires. You write down the desire that you did not reward, and how you felt as you let the emotion move through you.

When my brain thinks I really need something to survive, I have found it helpful to put my timer on and see how long that urge lasts.

Urges are comparable to little toddlers. When you take a toddler to the store, that toddler might see candy and ask for some. You say no. The toddler asks again and again. Then, they get louder and louder. What do many people do? They give the toddler the candy just to quiet them down. And this is exactly what we do with our urges.

The urges increase as we resist and avoid them. We give ourselves the little treat because we "have been on our diet for the past week now and deserve it." Our brain is sneaky and will convince us that we deserve the candy. But this does not serve our long-term goals.

Your small actions today create your future. Those little candies that don't melt in your hands, truly do melt into your mouth and eventually become a larger future problem. I only use this example because I tend to gravitate towards a quick handful of M&Ms whenever I see them. My brain wants me to believe that those little colorful beauties have some protein, so I should probably eat a few. We all need protein to survive, right!

We have to become detectives with our brain and find the lies that are so readily available.

The Urgent Desires Worksheet is the most simple way to break any habit, even those that are worn in and historical habits in your brain. They can be paved over and redirected to make more efficient pathways.

Just know, like the dogs, to expect more drooling at first, more discomfort and urges than ever before as you cover an old road and pave a new one. You can also expect to one day realize that you haven't thought about that old urge for a long time.

The drool will stop. The over-desire will be gone.

Ralph Waldo Emerson said, *"That which we persist in doing becomes easier, not that the nature of the task has changed, but our ability to do has increased."* This is exactly the point. We may always look at food and think, "Hmm, that looks good." The end.

What a "boring," but yet thrilling life. Wouldn't it be fulfilling to get that kind of control, that kind of power over yourself. You don't pretend that you don't want something, but rather, you acknowledge what you want, and just stop answering those urges until they really don't do anything for you anymore.

Instead of finding false or insatiable fake joy that comes from answering over-desires and urges, the challenge is to find true joy in our lives. Instead of living a numb life of false pleasures, you choose an intentional life that includes every emotion available.

Let's work on experiencing something other than numb. There have got to be more satisfying emotions. I promise you there are!

Do you wonder what joy in life is like instead of joy in food? Try this Urgent Desire Worksheet! This worksheet with help you start living a life of intention, long-term focus and satisfaction.

Urgent Desires Worksheet

100 ALLOWED URGES

When you have an urge, write it here instead of satisfying the urge. Then, start a timer to see how long the urge lasts. This is the best tool I use to break those unwanted habits. De-condition yourself by not answering 100 urges, and you will lose the over-desire for that habit. Here is a start to your new life.

Add a few more lines and you've got it!

_____

_____

_____

_____

_____

_____

_____

_____

_____

_____

_____

_____

_____

_____

_____

_____

_____

_____

_____

_____

_____

_____

CHAPTER THREE

5 Pillars to Permanent Weight Loss

"I want to know God's thoughts, the rest are just details"
-Albert Einstein

What every human likes is clarity. We want to know exactly what to do and what the reward will be if we do it. Even if the path is clear, that doesn't mean we will take the path. We just like knowing there is a clear path. Choosing to take it or not is not the point, right? Actually it is the point.

If you want any permanent change in your life, you must choose the path that leads to that change. The 5 Pillars to Permanent Weight Loss are those principles that will get you to the ideal health that you desire, and the weight that will provide you with maximum energy and enjoyment.

If you completed Phases I and II, then you already have some of the skills sets that are necessary for your lifestyle of permanent weight loss. You have learned some principles and created some great habits and thoughts, that will serve you on your journey of self-discovery.

Principles are fundamental truths that serve us. If you expected a step by step, food by food plan, then you will feel some disappointment right about now. I gave you some of that in Phase II, but for permanent weight loss, you must choose your own food plan from here on out.

This is similar to the former information I have provided. If you want to know what you should and shouldn't eat, there are many websites and books on the pros and cons of eating in specific ways and consuming specific foods.

I live by the idea that no one can tell me what is best for me. That information is for me to seek from my Creator, who I believe is God. He is the only One who can tell me how this creation, my body, will function at its peak. He created this "temple" that houses my spirit.

He is the only source of truth that I can 100% trust, who is looking out for my best interest at all times. He is the only One who showed up 100% for himself and that is what I am trying to learn to do for myself. So, if someone tells you that you are doing it wrong or that you are doing it right, always consider the source of all wisdom. Who do you trust with your life?

A protocol is a food plan that you will create based on reducing your body's insulin. Remember that insulin is a powerful hormone in your body that is responsible for storing fat.

There are five areas you will need to consider for your Protocol. Beyond that, you will apply the scientific method to discover more about you than you have probably ever known.

To know if you are making the wisest choice:
1. Go to The Source who for me, as I stated above, is God.

2. Answer the question, "Does it feel light?"

This just means, does the protocol you choose cause you to feel light physically, mentally, emotionally and spiritually? If so, then you must be onto something that is good for you.

And my ways are not your ways, so there is really no point telling you what I do, specifically. I can tell you that I continue to eat five small meals per day, whereas my master coach, Brooke Castillo, eats two meals. She seems to have plenty of energy and enjoys her lifestyle. I enjoy mine. I might change, but for now, this works well for me. Remember how I said this food plan would be simple and does not have to feel depriving? I am good to my word.

Let's take a quick look at the five pillars of permanent weight loss.

The Magic Formula—5 Pillars of Personal Permanent Weight Loss includes:
- Time Window

- What to Eat & What Not to Eat

- How Much to Eat

- When to Eat

- Documentation & Planning

Pillar #1: Time Window
When writing your personal protocol, I would suggest that you consider your time window first. What time do you like to wake up each day, when are you ready to go to bed at night?

What is the window of time that you feel comfortable choosing that will give your body the rest it needs from digesting food all day and allow time to repair your body during the night.

If you eat right before bed, sometimes your body spends valuable energy digesting rather than repairing. You may wake feeling tired, as if you did not get the rest your body truly needed and wanted. This is a debated idea and you can choose to believe it or not.

Consider the habits of your days and how they are serving your long-term goals. Some may choose to eat between 6:00am-6:00pm or you could choose to eat between 12:00 pm- 8:00pm. You get to choose!

Pillar #2: What to Eat & What Not to Eat
If you want to know what you should eat, then you just need to know that the minimum required foods for a human are vegetables, meat or beans, healthy fat, and water. Everything else is optional.

Basically, you should eat good quality protein and non-starchy vegetables with a healthy fat. When you say you need something to eat, those are the foods you are actually talking about. If it's truly hunger, then those are the food choices that will satisfy.

You know that just because you are giving up overeating, you certainly cannot give up all food. You only give up the foods that are causing you problems.

As you begin to become aware of the thoughts your brain likes to believe are true, but may not actually be true, you will find that your awareness of the foods you really want and don't want increases. Become in tune with how you feel. This is going to be key to choosing what types of foods you will eat.

Most of us buffer, or do things to avoid feeling any negative emotion. With food, if you have buffered for a long time, you probably don't know what your body actually likes and doesn't like. You just assume your body can tolerate anything.

What if you start looking to your body for answers as to what types of foods make you feel the most energetic--the most light? That seems simple, right? Yes, it is simple, but just like the de-conditioning worksheet with urges, it might take time for you to pave over old neurological pathways in order to open up your senses and receptors to create new pathways.

Our brain has delegated most of our eating to the subconscious level, so we just eat "on automatic." Remember that based on our old motivational triad, we are not going to want to change these habits because our brains believe that is a very inefficient use of our time and energy. So, be patient as you learn to uncover what your body truly likes to use for fuel.

We will talk more about concentrated foods soon, but just know, in general, you shouldn't eat flour, sugar, dairy (for some people) or processed foods. Why? Because our bodies aren't meant to consume these foods and they can create a lot of damage through inflammation and hormone imbalances.

Pillar #3: How Much to Eat
According to the information provided on all food packaging, we should understand that there are general guidelines for portion sizes. Are those boxes accurate? Actually, I really believe that your body will tell you what it needs. I have attached a Hunger Scale Worksheet related to this pillar in Chapter Four.

This worksheet will help you create and determine your own portion levels based on how you feel. Everything we do and don't do in life is because of a feeling. When we buffer with food, we eat more than we can use because we don't want to feel any negative emotion. When you can learn to feel the sensation of being full, then you will uncover what is really going on with your physical body.

Normally what's really going on with food has very little to do with food or your weight. Once you stop overeating, you may find you are left with emotions of disconnect from your spouse, loneliness, anger with a friend, self-loathing for past choices, pain from your past in general, or any number of other underlying issues that the food problem is just masking.

It's suffering on top of pain that we create for ourselves when we don't decide how much our body actually needs to feel satisfied. For example, after you overeat you feel uncomfortable. Then you might have a thought, "I shouldn't have eaten so much." This thought might create a feeling of disappointment. Thus, you feel physically full and mentally disappointed. You now have compounded the physical discomfort with a negative emotion.

This is a very important pillar of awareness. When you look at the Hunger Scale Worksheet in Chapter Four, you will be asked a few questions. The scale ranges from -10 to +10. The midline is when you are not hungry or full. A -10 is equivalent to starving, which most people in our country are not experiencing currently. And +10 is the stuffed feeling where you feel like that stuffed turkey that you just ate and you have to lean back in your chair and unbutton your jeans to make room for the pie about to be served. As you answer questions regarding this scale, you will be able to identify those thoughts about how you feel when you're eating.

Simply writing the range down and how it feels to you will create an awareness that can empower your results. You will want to ask yourself before, during and after you eat, "Where am I on the hunger scale now?" How does it feel to be at a -4?

How does hunger feel to you at a +8? These increments are small, but small and simple things create huge results! One more worksheet below is a Food Journal, where you simply write down every single thing you eat daily. Including all the licks, bites and tastes.

There are many phone apps that make this process convenient. I use one and love how easy it is to keep a record for my own accountability. Most people usually like to only record what they eat when they follow their protocol. That is not how change works.

For success to happen, you must be willing to fail. When reaching for a goal, success is always desirable, but failure is second best. Failure just means you are missing an expectation or a required action. Failure has nothing to do with a person's personal worth. When you fail at weight loss, that means you just need to figure out which piece of the protocol you are missing. If you don't obtain the weight you desire in the timeline that you set, this does not mean you are a failure.

Procrastination or quitting are the only non-useful results. So, fail, fail, fail some more and don't be afraid to fail. Most people will fail before they even really start, by quitting.

So they fail to try, out of fear that they might fail. Don't do this. You are capable of keeping a record of your actions in order to change your results.

I can promise you that the only reason you have negative results in your life currently is because you haven't taken the right action. You haven't learned the skill of failing. There is some expectation or required action missing. And guess what? That is the definition of failure. So don't ever be afraid to fail. If you had met all expectations and figured out the missing actions, then you wouldn't be reading this book. There is always something else to learn.

Pillar #4: When to Eat
Many past diets I have tried suggest 6 small meals. I pushed myself for a long time to fit in that 6th meal. I felt like I was forcing my mouth open, like we do with two year olds that shut their mouths to stop you from feeding them more.

Small children naturally know when they are done eating. If toddlers can stop eating when they are full, then what was I doing forcing my mouth open for that last small meal of the day? Somehow I thought if I followed someone else's plan exactly then I would look like they did in that little swimsuit.

I told myself, "If I can just get myself to keep eating then I will get that magic body!" What a crazy situation.

We do this to ourselves. We believe what others tell us is the best way. How others look would be so nice to experience ourselves. Why? Because we would rather be told exactly what to do, and then blame the process when it doesn't work, instead of learning how to process our uncomfortable emotions, face our underlying issues, and feel the consequences of our choices.

Becoming accountable to myself is a very inefficient action, according to my brain.

What does your brain think about you? Instead of forcing myself to eat, I decide what times I am going to eat in my time window (pillar #1). Simple. Do I feel better eating 6 meals or 2 meals? It's totally up to me!

Pillar #5: Documentation & Planning
Do not change any one of those 4 pillars unless you have given it two weeks. Can you change before two weeks? Of course! I am just suggesting you try to implement a protocol for two weeks before tweaking something.

Then, if you are not seeing the results you want, simply choose ONE pillar to change and make a change for two more weeks. This is precisely what the scientific method is.

You make an observation, such as, "I don't want to be 20 pounds overweight." Think of interesting questions, like, "I wonder how I could keep the weight off for good this time?"

Formulate a hypothesis, "Maybe if I cut out sugar and flour for two weeks, I will feel more energy. If I feel more energy, then I might move my body more. If I move more, then I might lose some extra non-useful weight and actually feel more energized. And, If I lose weight and feel increased energy then I will want to continue cutting out flour and sugar."

Gather data by keeping a food journal and checking in on the Hunger Scale to see how you are feeling. Then, you can either refine, re-assess, or reject the test altogether if you are not finding a general theme and positive result.

If you do not make a plan, then anything goes, including your waist. Record, tweak, plan, repeat. You got this! And yes, it really is that simple!

Be sure you create a protocol for yourself that you are willing to commit to. If the plan is unrealistic, then you will be using will power until you give up and decide it's not worth the effort.

Now part of the recording and documenting is really powerful when you add a record of your daily weight to the protocol. Seeing the number on the scale, daily, has some immediate negative thoughts for some people.

But, what if that number meant nothing about you as a human being of 100% worth? What if that was just a way to "check in" mentally to see where your weight is, daily.

Most of us will only want to write the number down if we approve of that number. What is approval? It's a feeling we get when we have a thought.

So, again, what is the thought you have when you look at the number on the scale. The only way it has any meaning is if you want to give it meaning. And that is exactly why this is a powerful addition to your protocol... daily, record the scale number. See what thoughts come up for you. It will be very insightful!

Until you uncover the underlying belief systems you have about yourself, you will continually fall back into old eating habits. Recording the number on a scale is a quick method to unveil what thoughts are holding you back and keeping you stuck at your current weight. Once you find the non-useful thoughts, then you can challenge those beliefs. As you take one thought at a time and re-direct it to be more useful, then your entire life trajectory will change. This is the lifestyle change you wanted, but didn't know how to create for yourself.

If you believe a scale has the power to make you feel sad or happy, then you are just confused. You get to decide what that number means to you every time. Period. It's what you decide that is causing any emotion. I encourage you to weigh yourself daily.

Practice this mental exercise of allowing a number to have no power over what you will think about yourself. It is just data for you. You can decide how to use that data.

"Hello" Scale Worksheet

Number today: (eg 20 lbs) _____

1. How do I choose to feel about this number?

   _____

   _____

   _____

   _____

   _____

   _____

2. What do I believe this number means?

   _____

   _____

   _____

   _____

   _____

   _____

3. What is the truth?

   _____

   _____

   _____

   _____

4. Could I peacefully own this number as a fact and not a statement about my life?

_____

_____

_____

_____

_____

_____

5. Describe what it feels like factually, and without judgement, to be in a body that weighs this number:

_____

_____

_____

_____

_____

_____

6. What can I choose to believe that is empowering?

_____

_____

_____

_____

_____

_____

7. What can I do to prove this belief system is true?

_____

_____

_____

_____

_____

_____

Food Protocol Worksheet

To create your own ultimate food plan that will lead to a healthy ideal permanent weight, answer these questions, record the data, and take massive action to repeat this process until you achieve your goals!

1. What is the beginning time and ending time of your daily eating window?

   _____
   _____
   _____
   _____
   _____
   _____

2. How many meals will you eat today?

   _____
   _____
   _____
   _____
   _____
   _____

3. What foods will you allow?

   _____
   _____
   _____
   _____

4. How much will you eat at each meal?

_____

_____

_____

_____

_____

_____

5. Document daily the number on the scale. Bi-weekly, assess your results and tweak one principle at a time until you have created the perfect protocol for your current body!

_____

_____

_____

_____

_____

_____

Food Journaling Worksheet

It's important to write down every single thing you eat daily. Include all bites and all licks

1. Write down everything you have eaten in the past 24 hours.

   _____

   _____

   _____

   _____

   _____

   _____

2. Make some notes on why you made the choices you did and how you felt, physically, throughout the day.

   _____

   _____

   _____

   _____

   _____

   _____

3. What is your ideal food journal? Write it below.

   _____

   _____

   _____

4. How do you imagine you will feel physically and emotionally when you make a habit of eating this way?

_____

_____

_____

_____

_____

_____

CHAPTER FOUR

Food Plan Bonus Material

"Good Inspiration comes from good information"
-President Russell M Nelson

It's Just Weight

Food is just that, food. Food is molecules on a plate. The number on a scale is just that, a number. Your weight is JUST WEIGHT. So why do we have so many issues around this number?

Why do we think that food has to make us feel good, emotionally, all the time? Did you know that food does not have the power to make you feel good unless you want it to?

The types of food you eat affects your brain chemistry.

We have talked about that. But what about the parties, the activities, the daily rituals?

Do those make us feel happy, content, sad or confused? No. Those situations cannot make us feel anything. They are neutral facts that are often outside of our control.

Circumstances in our lives do not inject sadness into some people and happiness into others.

If you think about it, the circumstances in our lives do not **cause** us any pain or joy. That does not mean we don't want to feel pain when we think about some of our circumstances but the pain *comes from our thoughts about the circumstances.*

The weather, the job, the kids, the spouse, your past and your weight are all circumstances. It can be proven in a court of law that you have 5 kids, a spouse, you grew up in Mesa, Arizona, your weight is 165 pounds, and the weather outside is currently 75 degrees. No one will argue with facts. There is nothing to argue about.

But look what happens when we add our own story based on our life filters to those facts. What happens when you add opinions and descriptions to situations. When you think, "Losing weight stresses me out," how does that feel? Probably stressful.

If you feel stressed, do you want to go eat salad? Most likely you will reach for something that numbs that stress down a bit, like a concentrated dose of something to stop that stressful feeling—maybe some dark chocolate or nachos. If you realize that those stressful thoughts are creating the emotions, then you get all your power and control back!

That, my friend, is some pretty amazing news! Knowing that there is no circumstance that can hurt you emotionally or mentally, allows you to take responsibility over your life and realize that you are in charge of how you will feel about any situation. The fact that you can also generate any emotion by choosing your thoughts is also one of my favorite tools to teach.

When you can separate the facts, or circumstances, from the thoughts you are having about those facts, then the awareness sets in and your prefrontal cortex lights up. The prefrontal cortex is the logical and long-term thinking part of your brain that looks out for your highest interest.

This is the area of the brain that you should always strive to allow your decisions to come from. Your primitive brain is similar to a toddler who wants everything right now, while your prefrontal cortex has been said to function better than any computer created currently in the world. This is the part that doesn't mind discomfort and is willing to use any amount of energy required to achieve a future goal.

So, as you separate the circumstances of your weight and the number on the scale, you can remind yourself that the number is just a number and the weight is "JUST WEIGHT." It has no power over how you will feel today if you don't want it to.

Drop the weight off your shoulders. Drop the weight off your mind. Focus on the reasons behind the weight: The evolution of survival instincts, the societal cues for feeling included in a group, the conditioning that happens from choosing to consume concentrated food and your brain's ability to make non-useful foods pretend to be extremely useful.

There is nothing wrong with you. You are perfect! You just haven't been given the skills necessary to handle the emotional and mental weight that comes when the physical weight is gone. The emotional weight loss feels just as threatening to your survival brain as the physical weight loss does.

Keep your brain in check by deciding what is a circumstance and what is just the story that you like to tell about your circumstance. This will be a burden lifted and a light in the darkness appearing before you, as you maneuver through this permanent weight loss path.

Circumstances vs. Thoughts Worksheet

Categorize the following. Circle if the following are (C)ircumstances or (T)houghts:

1. I love eating. C or T

2. Food brings me joy. C or T

3. The number on the scale is _____. C or T

4. My husband makes me happy. C or T

5. I have amazing legs. C or T

6. I am too busy to plan my food. C or T

7. I am a human. C or T

8. I am worried and overwhelmed. C or T

9. I hate my body. C or T

10. I have a lot of confidence. C or T

11. I am afraid to disappoint. C or T

12. I am ___ years old. C or T

13. My colleagues will accept me better if I were thinner. C or T

14. I have ____ color hair. C or T

Answer key: T, T, C, T, T, T, C, T, T, T, T, C, T, C

Do you notice there are lots more thoughts than circumstances? That is normal. Now you may choose to argue some of these answers, and that is exactly what you are allowed to do because you are human.
Enjoy!

Concentrated Foods: BUT I WANT THAT FOOD!

A little bit more about concentrated foods. Whenever I am working with clients, one of the first things they ask is, "Do I have to stop eating sugar and flour?" One of my favorite stories is of my older sister.

She was called by her husband and asked to prepare a dinner for his work colleagues.

My sister, we will call her Hailey, was trying to hurry home to get her house cleaned and food prepared for an unexpected gathering.

However, she didn't make it home for awhile. She was distracted by the cue associated with that big red sign with the red dot in the middle. Yup, the store of all stores-- Target. She found herself in the isles calling me.

I asked what she was doing and she said, "Oh well you know, if I am hosting a party in four hours, I need some new decorations, my house has such old stuff. I can't decide what table cloth cover to buy...grey or white?" I was listening curiously to how her brain continued down a path of buffering and seeking pleasure.

Suddenly, she was more concerned about picking out the right color of table cloth than getting her home clean and food prepared. She continued to walk the isles and I stayed on the phone. She went to get some popcorn because "it smelled so good."

And then "somehow she ended up in the dresses" because she "had nothing to wear." This story just got better and better. What goes with popcorn? Diet Coke of course. The clock was ticking, but Hailey's brain was working perfectly! Her brain was giving her plenty of ways to avoid the stress, feel lots of pleasure and use very little energy. She happily talked about the deals that were going on and how she didn't have any cute mustard colored dresses.

As she was walking toward the checkout lane to purchase her new home decor and dress for the upcoming party, she told me what was happening in her mind. She commented on how much better Diet Soda is with a candy bar. She went back and forth with thoughts of, "I shouldn't because we are going to Hawaii next week and I really want to look good in the swimsuit that I just bought. But it's just one candy bar, that is not going to make a difference. What will make the difference is the past few months, not just this one bar."

It was pure fascination to listen to her. Hailey even commented, "I am talking out loud to myself, so people around her probably think I'm crazy." She bought the innocent candy bar. The ultimate final moment was a re-cap later that evening.

The dinner went fine, but Hailey was so frustrated with her kids because when she had arrived home to re-decorate, clean and cook, they should have already had the home clean. She couldn't believe that she was going to have to do it all herself and nobody even cared. There was so much stress and so much anxiety building up.

The kids had no idea they were supposed to be cleaning instead of studying for school when Hailey got home. The kicker is, then Hailey had thoughts that created feelings of guilt. She offered the idea that she probably should have called her kids and told them she needed help instead of expecting them to know she would need help.

Okay, that was long, but perfect in every way to me. It is a story with very few facts, lots of drama, lots of self-generated stress and lots of concentrated foods to numb the stress (but in the end they compounded the stress). Those foods did not help Hailey get closer to achieving her body image goals. Hailey's story reflects exactly what our brains are programmed to do.

Do you see yourself in Hailey's story a bit? I do! We think we are crazy, but actually we are doing it all perfectly right. We are playing by the rules of evolution, society, our brain and our biology!

When a client asks if doing this "diet" will mean they have to let go of sugar and flour, I always say no. Just like I have stated already, it is not for me to tell you how to create your protocol. I have principles that work, and will give you information, but you must choose what you want to do with it.

President Russell M. Nelson of The Church Of Jesus Christ of Latter-Day Saints recently said, *"Good inspiration comes from good information."*

The more information gathered, the more you will want to test that information out and see if it works for you. Let me give you the basics regarding sugar and flour. Sugar and flour are concentrated foods.

It's like taking a grape, a natural source of food, and concentrating it into wine. The concentrated food artificially raises our insulin. The goal is to keep insulin low. Whenever we eat, insulin rises. If we are not eating, it drops. Insulin is released in response to any amount of glucose in the blood. Liquid sugar in soda is one of the main culprits of insulin excess.

Cutting out sugar and flour drops your insulin levels dramatically. By eating less often, you give insulin an opportunity to resensitize. Also, leptin and ghrelin start working and re-calibrate. When you eat concentrated foods, insulin rises quickly. Also, your body is unable to access the fat storage, so you will actually feel hungrier. How does this happen?

Your insulin actually blocks the leptin hormone so your brain cannot tell you if you're full. Remember that leptin tells your brain that you have some extra fat stores and don't need to keep eating constantly!

When that gets blocked, your brain is essentially kept out of the loop. You can eat a whole bag of chips and wonder if there are any more in the pantry. This is similar for ghrelin. Ghrelin tells you when you're hungry and when to stop feeling hungry. It is based on the volume and the fat in the food you eat. Refined or concentrated foods keep ghrelin from working properly.

Have you ever heard the phrase a "hollow leg?" I heard it from a teammate in college and wondered about it. She explained that it's where the food goes once your stomach is full. It wasn't until I learned the basics of these three hormones that I understood that the extra space isn't extra space at all. It's your brain playing hide-n-seek from yourself.

Insulin has wrapped a baby blanket over your brain, symbolically, like we do with babies. If they can't see us, they don't know if we are still there. Our brain is blocked from receiving the information needed to keep us feeling satisfied and healthy. We block our own receptors when we eat concentrated foods and by so doing, we can eat and eat and power through more food than anyone wants to admit.

That "hollow leg" has now moved to the other leg too. Learning to not block receptors is the key takeaway here. If you don't allow your mind to know what is happening, then you sabotage yourself from reaching your goals. You must keep your prefrontal cortex engaged in your food preparation and planning in order to maintain a healthy weight lifestyle.

You must keep your receptors open for leptin and ghrelin to do their jobs properly. This is where the Hunger Scale is most effective. You need to be able to actually feel what full feels like and when genuine hunger comes. Those are sensations that we don't want to block with concentrated foods and insulin spiking.

Hunger Scale Worksheet, Part 1

This is just a brief description of what you can do with this worksheet: If you really want to become aware of how you feel when you are eating, then I suggest writing the answers to the following questions for every interval. Basically, for optimum results you will want to stay between +3 and -3.

(-10)	(0)	(+10)
Starving	No feeling either way	Stuffed

1. Where are you on the hunger scale?

   _____

   _____

   _____

   _____

   _____

   _____

2. How does hunger feel to you at -4?

   _____

   _____

   _____

   _____

3. How does hunger feel to you at -8?

_____

_____

_____

_____

_____

_____

4. How much will you eat at each meal?

_____

_____

_____

_____

_____

_____

Giving Up Concentrated Foods Worksheet

If you choose to try living a life where your body is naturally receptive to what your hormones are trying to signal, then try this worksheet. Just answer the questions below:

1.   Do you want to become a person who doesn't eat concentrated food?

_____

_____

_____

_____

_____

_____

2.   What are the reasons that "clean eating" makes sense if you want to stop overeating?

_____

_____

_____

_____

_____

_____

3. What are the reasons this makes sense if you are trying to lose fat?

_____

_____

_____

_____

_____

_____

4. Write down all the reasons why it might be physically hard to give up sugar and flour.

_____

_____

_____

_____

_____

_____

5. Write down all the reasons why it might be hard, emotionally, to give up sugar and flour.

_____

_____

_____

_____

6. Have you been taught/conditioned that eating sugar and flour is normal? How?

_____

_____

_____

_____

_____

_____

7. Can you find some ways that it is abnormal to eat it sugar and flour?

_____

_____

_____

_____

_____

_____

8. How will you have to think about this differently if you want to lose weight and stop overeating?

_____

_____

_____

9. What habits do you have and what foods do you currently eat that will need to change in order to give up sugar and flour?

_____
_____
_____
_____
_____
_____

10. Which foods are the easiest to give up?

_____
_____
_____
_____
_____
_____

11. Which foods are the hardest to give up? Why?

_____
_____
_____
_____
_____
_____

Hunger Scale Worksheet, Part 2

This is a brief description of what you can do with this worksheet: If you really want to become aware of how you feel when you are eating, then I would suggest writing the answers to the following questions for every interval. **Fill this one out if you choose to eliminate concentrated foods: sugar and flour for six weeks.**

See how your responses differ from those on the Hunger Scale Worksheet, Part 1.

(-10)	(0)	(+10)
Starving	No feeling either way	Stuffed

1. Where are you on the hunger scale?

   _____

   _____

   _____

   _____

   _____

   _____

2. How does hunger feel to you at -4?

   _____

   _____

   _____

3. How does hunger feel to you at -8?

_____

_____

_____

_____

_____

_____

4. How much will you eat at each meal?

_____

_____

_____

_____

_____

Tedious Powerful Worksheet, Part 1

As often as you can handle it, use this worksheet. It's very tedious and time consuming, but the results are amazing. Sit down with this worksheet before you eat and document what you eat, in detail:

Pick a food you really like.

1.　　Name of food:

2.　　Quantity you want to eat:

3.　　Where are you on the hunger scale?

4.　　Describe the food in detail- look, smell, texture, color, etc.

5.　　Your feeling before eating the food:

6.　　Describe each bite and stop to write in between bites. Stop eating the food when you stop enjoying it.

- Describe the bite in detail:

　　　_____

　　　_____

- Describe the bite in detail:

　　　_____

　　　_____

- Describe the bite in detail:

  _____

  _____

- Describe the bite in detail:

  _____

  _____

- Describe the bite in detail:

  _____

  _____

- Describe the bite in detail:

  _____

  _____

- Describe the bite in detail:

  _____

  _____

- Describe the bite in detail:

  _____

  _____

7. Do all the bites taste the same? Circle One: Yes No

8. Does it start to taste less pleasurable or more pleasurable as you add bites? Circle One: Less More

9.   What is your feeling after eating this food?

_____

_____

10.   How much did you eat before you were satisfied?

_____

_____

11.   When did you stop eating?

_____

_____

12.   Where are you on the hunger scale after eating this food? How does this food feel in your body?

_____

_____

Tedious Powerful Worksheet, Part 2

After you have completed the Part 1 Worksheet, above, answer the following questions:

1. Did you overeat more when you were below zero on the Hunger Scale?

   _____

   _____

2. Were you able to feel more satisfied when you paid more attention to each bite?

   _____

   _____

3. How did your feelings affect the quantity of food you ate?

   _____

   _____

4. Were your before and after feelings the same or different?

   _____

   _____

5. Did you ever stop at bite one because you realized it wasn't something you wanted to eat?

   _____

   _____

CHAPTER FIVE

Confidence

"There are times when I just want to stay in bed all day, but I know that working out is the best way to get those endorphins going, which will make me feel better emotionally and physically."
- Heather Locklear

Regarding weight loss, our issues really are never about the weight. It's "Just Weight." Instead, our main desire is learning about understanding what truly satisfies and increases our confidence. Confidence is defined as being secure within yourself and your abilities.

Confidence is the ability to trust yourself, knowing you can experience any emotion (including failure) without being harmed. It's your overall opinion of yourself.

If confidence has to do with trusting yourself, then weight loss success has a lot to do with knowing that you will do what you say you will do. You will follow through on your protocol. You will take care of yourself despite feeling like you are too busy. And you will do the responsible and useful thing for yourself, even when you don't feel like doing it.

When I joined Weight Watchers with my sister about 10 years ago, I decided I wanted to lose about 20 pounds and then figure out how to keep it off. My sister lasted only a few months in the program. My dad also participated in this program and lost 100 pounds!

I am the only one of us who is still a member of that program. It would be really easy to stop going for the monthly check-in. I continue to "weigh in," not because I need to lose weight at this point, but because I understand the value of showing up for myself.

My husband has asked why I keep going. I tell him, like I tell myself, it's my accountability moment for myself. I want to see where my mind is. The number on the scale reminds me that what I am doing is still working. When that number rises, I can see where my thoughts are, what thoughts are useful regarding my weight and protocol, and which ones I can readily discard. The scale is a very easy accountability partner!

When I doubt my abilities, I feel the shift. I know that if can't count on myself, then I am not going to expect others to count on me. I also can't expect others to count on themselves when I cannot do the same.

When people say, "It is my husband's fault that I'm large. He cooks food, or wants to go out to eat every week." I think about all that power they are handing over to someone else or something else. They allow others to tell them how they should feel and what they should do and what kind of results they are destined to experience in life.

If you want to feel in control and self-confident, then you must start showing up for you. The ability to trust yourself starts from the consistent follow-through on your word to yourself. You are not born with confidence; you earn it by keeping your word to yourself and doing what you say you will do. This is the purpose of any protocol.

Be sure to only put into your protocol, those expectations that you plan to keep. The more you hold tight to what you write on your protocol, the more you will feel confident.

When you start to believe in yourself, you will see that those same skill sets will trickle into other areas of your life.

Confidence Scale

Confidence is what everyone wants, whether it involves food, performance evaluations, parenting, education, work, or any number of other areas in our lives. We want to feel confidence. Included below is also a great worksheet for weight loss or any area of your life! The -10 side of the spectrum includes thoughts such as, "I am so freakin' fat," "I'm not worth it," "It's useless to keep trying," "I will never be able to change," "I'm just a quitter."

When you use believable neutral thoughts about yourself to shift towards the middle-ground of curiosity, then you will find some hope and peace. Curiosity includes thoughts such as, "I wonder why my brain wants me to believe I'm not worth it," "I'm curious about why I feel like quitting," "It's interesting that I think I will never be able to change."

Once you are at this point, you will want to move toward more productive and useful thoughts, which will lead to more useful results. Examples include, "Maybe it's possible that I am worth it," "It's possible that I will succeed if I keep trying," "What if I choose to think that I'm not a quitter," "I am learning to become a person who is committed to seeing what is possible for me." These last thoughts lead to confidence and self-care, the +10 side of the scale. Try out your own ideas and see what you can create on your own confidence scale.

Confidence Scale Worksheet

(-10)	(0)	(+10)
Doubt/Self-Loathing	Curiosity	Confidence/Self-Care

1. Where are you on the confidence scale?

_____
_____
_____
_____
_____
_____

2. How does confidence feel to you at -4?

_____
_____
_____
_____
_____
_____

3. How does confidence feel to you at -8?

_____
_____
_____
_____

4. How much confidence will you need in order to reach your goals? Why?

_____

_____

_____

_____

_____

_____

CHAPTER SIX

Sensations and Feelings

"The Best Project you'll ever work on is you."
-Unknown

When we think about life, everything we do or pursue is because of a feeling we hope to have. Truly the worst part of life is an emotion. Emotions are what make life bad and good. If we knew we could handle any feeling, then our confidence would be endless and our willingness to fail and succeed would thrive.

We take the fear out of experiencing life when we allow ourselves to feel anything! So, if feelings are why we do everything we do, then we need to know what the difference is between a feeling and a sensation.

Sensations:
Sensations are involuntary and start in the body. They are a direct experience with life.

When you are hungry, the hormone ghrelin sends signals to your brain to tell you that you should probably go get some fuel. And then, leptin will tell you when you have the physical sensation of being full.

Your stomach may growl and you may experience some waves of hunger. When you are thirsty after doing some intense yard work in the summer, your body reminds you to go get some water.

What about when you have an injury? You body sends signals to the brain that something is not right and action may be required. Heat, cold, hunger, thirst, and pain are all examples of sensations. They start in the body and move to the brain.

Feelings:
Every feeling we have is caused by a thought. Thoughts always create feelings! They start in the brain and move into the body. They are vibrations we feel from chemicals being released, and these emotions are in a variety of places and intensities in our bodies.

These vibrations are what we describe as emotions or feelings. Feelings are voluntary and start in the brain. When we satisfy our sensations with food, ghrelin and leptin inform our receptors that we are full. However, our survival brain fabricates cravings even after we feel satisfied.

You are not hungry, but your brain believes that those concentrated foods are what keep you alive. You have conditioned yourself to begin releasing dopamine as soon as dinner is over, in preparation for dessert. Until you finally eat a dessert, that urge to eat more will persist.

You know, logically, that you are full or at least satisfied, but what about that urge? Remember that we talked about the dogs that drool? If we want to see what it actually feels like to live a full human life experience, then we must be willing to feel it all.

There is a difference between the bodily sensation of hunger as well as the feelings we have about hunger. We eat for both reasons and it is just an interesting opportunity for all of us to become watchers, or outside observers, of our own brains to see what is actually happening when we are eating.

Your motivation for everything you work so hard to achieve comes because of the way you think you will feel once you reach your goal. When you truly think about your compelling reason for trying to lose weight, most likely you really want to feel healthy, energized, beautiful, young, and adequate--for yourself and sometimes for others as well.

The most incredible part of understanding that your thoughts generate every emotion is that you do not have to wait for that weight loss in order to feel energized, beautiful, young, adequate and healthy. If you realize your innate power, you also realize that your weight is JUST WEIGHT and has no power over you. Then you no longer have to wait for the feeling that you are working so hard to achieve.

Accomplished and successful feelings can be yours to enjoy during the journey to your ideal weight. Working on a goal from an inner feeling of abundance makes it easier to achieve your desired outcome, especially when obstacles are ahead. You already feel amazing, so what is a boulder in your path? It will take just a few moments for you to learn what other amazing skills you have inside that you can use to conquer a boulder.

Processing Emotions

When we talk about emotions, most people were never taught in school what to do with them. This is something that would be great for you to teach your kids so they will be that much further ahead in their mental and emotional health when they are our ages.

There are three things most humans do with any emotion:

#1. Resist
#2. React
#3. Avoid

What we need to learn to do is:

#4. Allow

Resist

When we resist an emotion we can liken that action to holding a beach ball down in the water. The more we push it away, the more pressure and tension is built up. Or the idea that you are pushing against a closed door that wants to open. The emotion intensifies the more you resist. It may feel constricting, like you cannot take a full breath.

Reacting

Reacting to an emotion typically looks like crying, yelling or screaming. Sometimes you think that this actually makes your situation better. You yell at your spouse or kids because they don't help with house cleaning or they don't do whatever it is you expect them to do. If they do what you ask them to do after you yell, then unfortunately, you think you have won and are now in control. This confirms your thought error that all you have to do is get mad and everything will fall into order. However, this is not the lasting emotion you want. Instead of processing an emotion, you just act them out. Yelling is only a temporary relief from the built up tension of resisting that emotion.

Avoid
Humans naturally want to feel pleasure. We avoid negative emotions by acting in ways that numb us to negative feelings. This is easy today. We have concentrated foods that take that edge off of overwhelm and stress. We avoid feeling a negative emotion by overeating, over-drinking and overworking. These are the most common, but there are many other ways to numb us from negative emotions.

When we feel stressed, it seems easier to pretend there isn't a problem and avoid the stress by eating food as a solution to end the problem. That action of eating, which came from a negative emotion, does not solve the cause of the problem.

Allowing an Emotion
In order to really feel an emotion and gain the benefits of unlimited self-confidence, then you must choose option #4. Allowing an emotion looks and feels like opening the door to that resistant feeling. It feels like you can breathe again, even if its a negative emotion. It's choosing to feel instead of react, and not to eat instead of avoiding a negative emotion. When you allow emotions, then the true problems unveil themselves.

You are choosing to feel discomfort, boredom, worry, loneliness, fatigue and restlessness. Your primitive brain is working and blaring a red light with a huge neon sign that says, "Warning, turn back, get some sugar now! You could die if you do not return to the safety of your couch!"

Allowing negative emotion is also called "choosing to feel it." Stop running away with your popcorn, soda pop and chocolate when you have a lot to get done, and overwhelm and busyness set in.

All of us experience pain. That's just part of being human.

Here are the steps to process pain or negative emotions:

1. Something happens or happened that triggered your pain.

2. You can't make sense of it.

3. You feel intense emotional discord, which just means the vibrations in your body caused by the thoughts are painful.

4. At this point, you either resist, react, or avoid....or allow.

5. Don't resist, react, or avoid, just allow. Say to yourself, "This is (whatever the emotion is). I can handle this." Then seek to find it in your body, describe it, and welcome it as a part of your life.

Self-discovery is a fun way to look at this weight journey.

CHAPTER SEVEN

Choose Your Emotion

"Strength doesn't come from what you can do. It comes from overcoming the things you once thought you couldn't."

-Nikki Rogers

There is a tool called the Silver Platter that we use to help clients understand which feelings they choose to avoid and which ones they tend to prefer. If you were at a nice social function and you saw waiters walking around with silver platters on their hands offering hors d'oeuvres--which ones would you choose?

Now think of these silver platters covered with emotions to offer you. The waiter asks you to go ahead and enjoy some emotions. Which emotions would you choose? Most people think they would only choose the positive emotions, but this is not what life is about.

As a member of The Church of Jesus Christ of Latter-Day Saints, I believe there is "opposition in all things." (Book of Mormon, 2Nephi 2:11) When someone dies, we think thoughts that generate sadness, sorrow, and grief. We don't always want to feel happy. When we resist, react and avoid all the negative, then we are also avoiding the good stuff in life.

You cannot understand the positive without the negative. So, why do we think we need to be happy all the time? I would offer that maybe we can't and don't want to always be happy. When we are not happy, we eat so that our neurological receptors are dulled to the negative emotional pain.

When we think we are happy, we think we know what "happy" truly is. And yet, without the unhappy feelings, there is no full understanding of true happiness. Denying feelings is what I call living on the outskirts of your life. When you continually avoid negative feelings, then you are by default, missing out on what the other side feels like.

If you choose to take happiness, peace and self-confidence off the silver platter, then you are essentially also asking to understand what unhappy, chaos, and self-doubt feels like. Only then will you truly be able to feel happy, peaceful and self-confident.

So many of us are missing out on the best part of our life because we are afraid of what the negative emotions might feel like. Our brains tell us to run away. But what if you just stopped, stood still and felt the negative emotion?

If those emotions are just created by your own thoughts, and are vibrations in your body, then you can handle them. They will not hurt you. Your brain gets confused and cannot differentiate between real and false fear. It is just doing it's job, and you can challenge its usefulness in your life today.

Four Core Human Fears

When it comes to weight loss, we have discussed that most of our weight loss goals have very little, if anything, to do with the actual weight. Once we lose that weight, then we are still left with our brains.

What is it that brought you to be overweight in the first place? It is over-hunger and over-desire. One of the reasons we repeat these weight loss cycles is because we do not manage our minds. Once the weight is gone, then we are left to deal with the other problems we see in our lives. Because most of those underlying concerns have to do with even more unpleasant emotions, we go back to eating to get away from our negative emotions. At least, eating is somewhat controllable.

There are four core fear-based beliefs that most humans have. These fears hold us back from making permanent change!

I think you should all understand that most of us really don't want to lose weight. Most people would rather eat whatever they want to eat and somehow magically maintain the perfect figure. Whatever you think the perfect figure is, it will be right for you. My perfect figure will not look like your perfect figure.

But what we do have in common is that we really don't want to watch calories and worry about what we can and can't eat. We want an ideal healthy weight that will carry us into old age without having to worry about food at all.

We also have been socialized to believe that if we are not thin, then we are not good enough. And, if we don't eat that birthday cake, then we are rude and, again, something is wrong with us.

These two actions, eating cake and being thin, are not compatible for most humans.

I wonder if those that are thin in their work related-careers (i.e., models), don't wish they could stop worrying about food and what they can and can't eat.

During the holidays we are going to want to partake of all the goodness that is being baked. The aroma of cinnamon and sugar fills the air and we love the smell of raising white bread and pumpkin rolls.

Why is yummy food such a draw? What if you just didn't have a desire for those foods at all. Is that even possible?

It is possible. We discussed the process of how to get rid of the over-desire for foods that don't serve your body well in Chapter Two.

Here are a few tips about the emotion of fear that will help you become more aware of your brain's cleverness as you continue to work to de-condition yourself from your over-desire for food.

Fear is a typical daily experience for most of us. And what do we fear?

There are four core fears that most of us have:
1. Fear of not being good enough

2. Fear of missing out on life

3. Fear that you don't have that "thing" needed to be happy

4. Fear of not being liked

Let me show you what I mean when it comes to weight loss. If you were choosing to believe the thoughts from fear number one, then you might think that there is something wrong with you, that you should know how to lose weight and keep it off. Maybe you shouldn't bake cookies before you eat your planned meals because you know you do not have enough willpower to resist eating the whole batch. Or, maybe you know you are an intelligent woman that just has no control. And the list goes on.

What other ideas come to your mind when you think about why the underlying fear that you might not be enough comes into play? What about the idea that if you were just your ideal weight then everything else in life would be so much easier?

Did you know that once you get to your ideal weight, your brain is still there with you, telling you that you are not enough....just in a different area of your life. As Brooke Castillo says, *"You can't hate yourself thin."*

Nobody likes to talk about loving themselves. Either people think that talking about love is a waste of time or that they already know the information and don't need any more self-love for whatever the reason. People think love is fluffy. But actually, unless you learn to feel love inside first, then losing weight will be an uphill battle!

Now if you are choosing to believe the lies from your brain about missing out on life, then you might be thinking thoughts like: If I was thinner, my husband would want to take me on that vacation to Hawaii. I am missing the vacation of my dreams because of my weight. Or, maybe it's the idea that if you could just figure out your weight issue, then you wouldn't yell at your kids so much and your relationships would be deeper and more satisfying.

Because you are overweight, you may believe that you cannot connect with your kids as easily. So, you think you are missing out on relationships with your kids due to your weight issues.

It doesn't matter what the excuse is, your brain wants you to believe that you are not enough and your weight is the cause of your missing out on life.

This just isn't true.

The reason we want anything is because of how we think it will make us feel.

This is why learning to generate a love for yourself is so important. How can you take care of your family if you don't even like you? How can you lose weight and keep it off if you are self-loathing?

How can you feel the enjoyment of life if you are not allowed to feel joy until you are the perfect size. And not only that, but like I said earlier, once you are the perfect size, you will just find something else to hate-- maybe the saggy skin left behind.

Learning to believe in yourself, believing that you are good enough and that there is nothing you are missing and there is an abundance of love, will change your weight loss process. You need to challenge your brain when it offers the idea that you are not enough.

You want to challenge your brain when it tries to convince you that you might miss something great if only you were a few pounds less. Don't trust your brain. You are not your brain. You are an amazing, thriving and wonderful person with unlimited potential. The perfect weight will never make you feel that truth.

What about fear number three--the fear that you might not have what everyone else has? If you had "that thing" then you would be happy. If you had her hair, their home, that car and lived in that city, then you would be happy.

And then finally, fear number four: If you don't have those things and are not thin enough, then people won't like you. If you are not liked, then what is the point of all this hard work? Do you see the dilemma in these fears?

Do you see how they hold you back from enjoying your authentic and human self? Try to notice how these fears have played out in your past weight loss goals. They are common and constant.

The Cause of All Your Problems and the Solution!

Most people seeking to lose weight are waiting for that special new food plan, the action plan. They are striving to find out what they need to DO to FEEL better. But this is backwards.

We cannot DO anything to FEEL any better. That is not the way to achieve permanent weight loss.

What we eat is caused by a feeling-- we eat because we feel lonely, tired, sad, bored, or any other emotion. We don't eat and then feel lonely, sad, bored or tired. Those feelings can be compounded by eating, but eating does not cause the emotion.

You now know that the problem with weight is just your thoughts about your weight. The emotions you feel are caused by your thoughts. Those emotions drive all of your eating.

When you eat too much, then the result you get is that you become overweight. It's that simple.

If the result you want is to not be overweight, but rather keep a healthy and energetic weight, then what do you have to do? What is that magical action plan that all who are reading this book have been waiting for? The action plan is the individual protocol.

If you are very detailed and learn to trust yourself with what you have written on your personal protocol, then you will succeed. In order to take the massive action on your protocol, what will you need to feel? Maybe you will need to feel commitment or courage, drive or discomfort?

In order to generate these types of emotions, what would you have to think? I have found helpful thoughts range from: "I am willing to do what it takes to succeed this last time," "I can do hard things", "Today I will choose to honor my protocol" and "I am worth taking care of."

Any of these types of thoughts might generate the drive and courage needed to follow through with your protocol and continually try new pieces until you get the result you want.

Neutral Thought Method
Sometimes we just don't believe we are capable or good enough to enjoy lasting results. If this is you, then why not try a tool I teach called the Neutral Thought Method. This is a way you can go from total self-doubt, "I am unable to lose weight," to complete self-confidence, "I totally got this!"

Take baby steps towards your goal thought. Your "goal thought" is a thought that you believe 100%. If you believe a thought 100%, then you already have the result you seek. If your thoughts are what drive your results, then those thoughts are going to need to be believable!

If you are at a -10 on your confidence scale, then what kind of thoughts will move you, or bridge those thoughts towards the +10 side of that scale. It's like climbing up a ladder one step at a time until you finally reach the ultimate, unicorn thought that, at first, your brain rejected as a possibility for you!

Try these few and then think of more that you can work on:

- I used to believe I was _____, but now I am learning to believe I am _____.

- I have a human body and this is a human stomach and these are human legs.

- I am a human and all humans are flawed.

- I am a human and it's possible that I am enough.

- I'm looking forward to believing that I am amazing.

- It's possible that I am amazing at some things.

- It's possible that I am amazing.

- I am amazing.

Can you see the progressive thought process. You must find believable thoughts along your road to permanent weight change. As you believe these thoughts, your level of belief will show in your results.

How Do You Want To Feel Today Worksheet

1. What are the feelings you choose?

    _____

    _____

    _____

2. Imagine a Silver Platter of emotions. What are the ones you need? What are the ones you want to feel on purpose? (Remember to include both positive and negative)

    _____

    _____

    _____

3. Name three positive emotions you want:

    _____

    _____

    _____

4. Name three negative emotions you don't want, but need:

    _____

    _____

    _____

5. Name three emotions that are not useful (whether you want them or not). Sometimes we think worry, confusion, doubt, overwhelm and other emotions are necessary when actually they only hold us back from progressing towards our goals:

_____

_____

_____

CHAPTER EIGHT

Self-Care

"You can't hate yourself thin."
-Brooke Castillo

Over and over again, I work with clients on their self-care. Did you know that the Bible states that we are to obey God's word. Guess what God has told us? "Thou shalt love the Lord thy God with all they heart, and with all they soul, and with all thy mind. This is the first and greatest commandment. And the second is like unto it.

*"Thou shalt love thy neighbor **as thyself**."*

Do you see what that commandment said? It says to **love yourself**.

Most moms that I talk to tell me (in fact, I heard it again this morning), that the kids are #1. They come before her self-care, always. Mom's simply glide over the last part of the commandment and feel totally justified because they are *"helping others."*

If you wait for the conditions to be perfect to take care of yourself, you'll never start. Others will always take priority over your physical, mental, and emotional health.

There would be no reason for discussion about this priority if we waited for perfect conditions. Conversation closed.

But, what if we really thought about what God commanded us? What if we could truly love our neighbors based solely on our ability to feel love?

Loveability has nothing to do with you. Loveability is about the person who is loving you. Your ability to be loved is never about you. You are already 100% loveable and of infinite worth. Other people's capacity to love determines their ability to love, not our lovability.

Are you truly capable of loving others if you do not know what love for yourself feels like? When you continually neglect your own self-care, how do you feel? If you feel tired and overwhelmed, exhausted and frustrated with all the required busyness of life, how do you show up for your kids? When you neglect your physical, emotional, mental and spiritual health long enough, you will begin to atrophy in some areas.

As an athlete, I recall breaking a bone in my foot. I had to wear a boot for just a few weeks. When the boot came off, not only did it look terrible, but the muscles had atrophied. I was shocked at the rapid loss in muscle mass. How do we regress so quickly? It's simple. When we neglect any area of our life, the primitive brain steps in to be efficiently inefficient.

If you are not diligently caring for your own health, you will find that when your kids have grown and gone, not only might they do the same and neglect themselves, but you may be left with consequences that are not going to serve you to help you become the best version of you. Those practiced rituals that you lived for so long will need to be re-wired in your brain.

Instead of not having enough time to plan meals, feel emotions and exercise, you actually need to start by putting these things in your schedule every day. Plan to put yourself first.

Here are a couple examples to help you understand the importance of taking care of yourself so you can take care of your family and others. First is the idea that if a plane were to have an emergency crash landing, the flight attendants always advise that parents put the oxygen masks on themselves before they put the masks on their kids. Another one is the idea that you cannot pour any love from an empty pitcher. This makes complete sense.

But, then again, we logically know many things that we just don't do, even though applying those things could help us evolve into a better version of ourselves.

Change is the key to life. You must be learning, changing and experiencing in order to feel all that life has to offer. The tricky part of always giving is that at times, you are rewarded for serving. The reward comes from external sources that validate your thoughts toward continuing to give despite neglecting your own needs.

You are viewed as the giver. But you don't give to yourself, so you are starving for some attention from you. This internal need is often reflected in the outward action of buffering with food and the result is being overweight.

Our spirits and bodies need our attention too. You are #1. You are the most important person that you can take care of. You cringe at this statement because it goes against serving your neighbors. Do not forget the second half of the second greatest commandment, *"Thou shalt love thy neighbor as thyself."*

If you cannot love yourself, then you will eventually feel worn out, burdened, and bitter because you will feel that there is always one more need that you must fill.

That one more need to be filled, will be filled so much easier and with a deeper sense of love if you fill your own vessel first. Do not neglect yourself. If you want to be the best mom to your kids, show them how to take care of themselves and then serve others, by first taking care of yourself.

You can tell your kids to be kind to themselves, to say only positive words, and to enjoy life, but what they see from you is a much louder example of your priorities than your words. Be your own best friend. What would you say to your friend that is constantly giving and continually feeling worn out?

Think about where you find your joy in life. If you typically find most of your joy in food, think about what might happen if you spent that joy learning what you love and then loving others. Do not ever sacrifice healthy eating or sacrifice your emotional health for anyone else. Your kids need you to be healthy.

The beautiful part of living the second greatest commandment fully is that your energy will increase, your confidence will expand and your love will include more people than you were able to serve in your self-neglected state.

Most food we eat is insatiable, you can never get enough. Eating the food that your body needs will satisfy. When it comes to relationships, money, confidence, time, and contribution, the most satisfying parts of life come from challenging your primitive brain.

True joy will come from choosing to embrace the discomfort inevitable for change and from using energy until you achieve the results you want. Satisfaction can be found only internally and not from anything outside of you. J-O-Y is a Journey Of You. Personal weight loss is a self-discovery process. Change your mind first and the body will follow.

Joy Worksheet

1. What are your top five sources of joy?
   a. _____
   b. _____
   c. _____
   d. _____
   e. _____

2. How do you feel about this list?

   _____
   _____
   _____

3. Do you need to diversify more?

   _____
   _____
   _____

4. What would you like your top source of joy to be?

   _____
   _____
   _____

5. In what ways can you create joy internally. Give two examples.

   _____
   _____
   _____

Self-Appreciation Worksheet

Make a list of all the things you like and appreciate about yourself. They can be small things or big things. Please write down at least 12 things:

1. _____

2. _____

3. _____

4. _____

5. _____

6. _____

7. _____

8. _____

9. _____

10. _____

11. _____

12. _____

CHAPTER NINE

5 C's to Change

"Wake up with determination. Go to bed with satisfaction."
- Unknown

5 Quick Steps Toward Permanent Change

I want to end with one quick tool as you work to achieve your "impossible" goal of permanent weight loss and lifetime health. You have a desire to achieve a healthy ideal weight as a lifestyle instead of a recurring daily battle. I only say "impossible" because your survival brain is going to tell you that it's impossible. If you already decide that it's impossible, then there is nothing stopping you from going all out on yourself. Therefore, your survival brain won't have any good arguments.

What's there to lose? You can always go back to your old habits and hold on to all the unwanted weight. That is an option available anytime during this process. Your old thoughts will produce your current results. You always have that choice. But if you know there is no way you will actually figure it out this time, then there is no fear of failure, just pure curiosity to see if this program actually works.

These tools might be the missing pieces of the weight issue that have cost you so much wasted time, money and energy. If you use these tools, you can maintain a healthy weight that will allow you to enjoy more time with your family and more success in your future goals.

What if this program works? What if it is possible? The fact that your brain created a goal for you instantly means there is a possibility. **What do you think?** That's all that matters.

Here are the 5 C's to Change:
1. **Compelling Reason**: What do you want and Why? If you don't know why, then your goal won't stick.

2. **Commitment**: You must believe 100% that you are going to continue to reach for your goal, especially when your brain says it's too hard; you are not good enough; if you spend too much time going for this goal, then you will miss out on something of more importance; or, even if you do reach it, someone will still not accept you. Plan for these lies and move forward anyway. You've got this!

3. **Courage**: This emotion will come as you commit and recommit daily, to YOU. It will require courage to take the massive action towards your goals. Know that massive action just means you don't stop until you get that result! Even if you have tried "everything," there is still something else you can try!

4. **Capabilities**: This is the skill set you learn from focusing on one goal at a time. You want to lose weight? Do it! You now have the education and

tools to make that happen permanently. Once you learn how to show up for yourself consistently in the area of weight loss, then use those same skills in other areas that feel hard and overwhelming, like your relationships, your money or your time management. You are gaining capabilities that you can apply to other areas of your life once you have mastered one area.

5. **Confidence**: Lastly, the coveted confidence--the word that most people want more of. This doesn't come without effort. The more you learn to trust yourself, the more confidence you will achieve. Confidence is the result that many moms I work with say they want. It's not only possible, but small practices yield immense confidence that can be found no other way but through the fire of discomfort. Confidence is yours for the taking. So take it! Permanent weight loss is just another way of saying, "confidence gained"! Belief creates self-confidence. Stay committed to your beliefs and confidence will be your happily ever after.

CHAPTER TEN

Final Words

"What I know for sure is this: The big secret in life is that there is no big secret... There's just you, this moment and a choice."
-Oprah Winfrey

The word "busy" gets in the way of many dreams these days, especially when it comes to weight loss. Many of my clients feel very "busy." Now that you know what you can do with emotions, and that emotions are created by your thoughts, I want to encourage you to choose a more useful word. Choose a word that feels invigorating instead of burdensome.

Maybe the top three emotions that you might choose from that silver platter could be: intentional, driven, and open...open to inspiration that will come continually throughout your days if you allow it! Remember, "busy" is just an emotion created by a thought. If you want to identify with being a "busy person" by all means, go ahead. But, if you find that "busy" doesn't feel good, then you have the power to change. You might invite thoughts that create more intentional, driven, and open feelings, such as: "I do have time to plan healthy food" or "I am capable of honoring my protocol," or "food is just molecules on a plate that my body needs to live the best version of me—they don't have any power over me," or "I am learning to believe I am a person who is able to trust myself." See how those sentences feel. Make up your own. Create the euphoric feeling you think weight loss will give to you, right now!

You don't have to wait to be the right weight in order to feel amazing today! You already are amazing. You just have to believe it and then you will feel it. Weight loss is so much easier if you already love and accept yourself.

I want to leave you with a few empowering beliefs for you to "try on" as you work through your neutral thoughts towards full belief in yourself. Enjoy!

- What others think about me is 100% about them.

- I was made for this.

- Fear is no big deal.

- I am capable.

- The worst that can happen is a feeling.

- I have my own back.

- Failure earns success.

- The better I fail, the more confident I am.

- Busy only pretends to be necessary.

- What I make my weight mean about me is the worst or the best that can happen.

The tools in this book are meant to be used. Applying the tools will be the difference between this book being "just another weight loss book" and "the book that made all the difference" for you. Understanding and reading is great, but applying is where the magic happens.

Stop ignoring your own needs and start living the best version of you. There is no reason to keep that extra weight and there is no reason to be unhappy. Don't find comfort in a content life. Be curious about what more is out there just waiting for you. Give yourself the gift of taking care of you this year and see what kind of impact that has on the world around you.

It will feel uncomfortable, I'm not going to lie, but the transition of trusting yourself will be the best gift you can ever give to your family. They will see how creating an extraordinary life is done. Let's not worry about your weight or what you should or shouldn't eat ever again. It will take practice, just like learning a new sport.

You have to first learn the rules, then start playing the game in order to get more comfortable with the sport. It's the same for yourself and weight loss. Learn what the rules are that your primitive brain plays by, then see what the prefrontal cortex offers.

Then it will be time to decide, intentionally, which team you will choose to play for? You are the referee. You are both sides of the game. You determine the outcome of the score. What will it be this time?

I want to share with you something I realized while writing this book. I pondered on what most people want when it comes to another weight loss plan.

Do you know what I was told by my clients? "Just tell me exactly what to do." That is the plea of many of my clients.

They ask, "Please just tell me how to lose weight, how to feel better, how to increase confidence in myself, how to get more hours in my day, or how to have more energy to get through the things on my never-ending to-do list."

Phase II tells you specifically a protocol you can use to lose weight. It is the phase that tells you what you think you want. I feel like this is what the "Old Testament" was for the Jewish people. They believed that if they were told exactly what to do, then they would get to the "promised land."

For this book, if I tell you exactly what to do, then will you have that permanent weight loss you so desire? What if that is not what you really want?

When parents tell their kids exactly what to do, the kids often feel resentful and frustrated. The kids will blame their parents when their lives don't turn out the way they were told it would be.

One of my clients recently told me, "I think if you told me exactly what to do, no matter what you told me, I probably wouldn't consistently do it. And then I would feel like I'm falling short. That is what I feel about most things in my life-- I fall short of what I should be doing or could be doing." When we are told what to do in every part of our life, we feel controlled.

The beautiful part of life is that we have free agency. If we are supposed to feel joy and be happy, but are also made aware that there will be "opposition in all things" (Book of Mormon, 2 Nephi 2:11), then how do you reconcile the contradiction?

You don't. There is opposition in all things SO THAT you can feel joy and happiness.

You learn by making mistakes. The more mistakes you make, the closer you will get to that perfect, permanent weight loss that you so desire.

You get to decide what is best for you. I told you in Phase II what I think is best for you, but that has nothing to do with you. That is a plan that works well for me.

What works for you? Phase III is about self-discovery and using your agency to choose for yourself what is best for you. You are learning to trust yourself.

As I explained in the Introduction, learning to trust yourself is the hardest part of any plan. Making a plan and sticking to it will create confidence that is limitless. It doesn't really matter what the food plan is if you aren't abiding by it. I can make you an amazing food protocol and you can make yourself an incredibly effective protocol, but it's useless if you don't use it.

Phase II states what you think you want— a strict food protocol.

Phase III tells you what you really want. It's the "New Testament" way. It's a higher way of living. Self-reliance and personal inspiration is what you really want. It is the ability to learn how to show up for yourself, and trust that you know what to do for yourself better than anyone else does. Phase III is simple, but it's scary and takes a lot of faith because the responsibility is on you. However, with the Lord's help, "nothing...is impossible" (St. Luke 1:37).

Learning to trust your own intuition is more powerful than any given "food plan." While your primitive brain is designed for survival, your indomitable divine spirit desires deeper meaning and purpose. Being the creator of your life is part of the purpose of life.

This is the challenge we all have. Stop. Be still. Listen. What is your body telling you? What do you need right now? What feels true to you? ...then, go with that and you can't go wrong.

Remember, it's Just Weight! You've got this!

∞∞∞∞∞∞∞∞∞∞∞∞∞∞∞∞∞∞∞∞∞∞

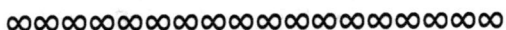

Thank You for Reading this book!
Congratulations on your desire to work on a
healthy weight lifestyle.

About the Author

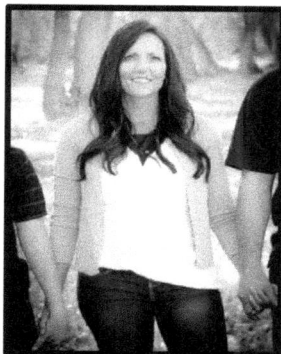

Amy Twiggs is a wife and a mother of four teenagers. She is also certified as a Life & Weight Loss Coach. She equips and empowers her clients to enjoy more control and satisfaction in their lives on their journey of unveiling their personal potential to themselves. Thus, her greatest joy is to help you find yours. Amy helps you take a closer look at your belief systems and how those thoughts are creating your current results. She is a former elite gymnast and in 1993 she was a member of the developmental National Women's Gymnastics Team. She received a full-ride athletic scholarship for gymnastics from Stanford University where she obtained a Bachelor's Degree in Psychology with a focus in Health & Development. Amy's education has provided many opportunities for her to give back and she looks forward to serving you.

If you want help applying these **Weight Loss Tools**, you can contact Amy by going to AmyTwiggs.com or FlippinAwesomeCoaching.com